Front Line of Defense

The Role of Nurses in Preventing Sentinel Events

Foreword written by Sally Sample, RN, MN, FAAN

Joint Commission Resources Mission

The mission of Joint Commission Resources is to continuously improve the safety and quality of care in the United States and in the international community through the provision of education and consultation services and international accreditation.

Joint Commission Resources Educational programs and publications support, but are separate from, the accreditation activities of the Joint Commission. Attendees at Joint Commission Resources educational programs and purchasers of Joint Commission Resources publications receive no special consideration or treatment in, or confidential information about, the accreditation process.

For more information about Joint Commission Resources, please visit our Web site at *www.jcrinc.com.* For more information about the Joint Commission on Accreditation of Healthcare Organizations, please visit *www.jcaho.org.*

Table of Contents

Foreword

"Influence gained is not by preaching, but by what we are...be heroic in your every day's work." Florence Nightingale (1820–1910)

Nurses are—and have always been—concerned advocates for the quality of care. Every nurse feels a responsibility for the people in his or her care. Nurses strive to provide a safe, nurturing environment and to be clinically competent in applying nursing skill and therapeutics. In today's turbulent health care environment, nurses often comment that they work in an environment of "near misses." Due to their continuous vigilance, nurses often catch potential errors or sentinel events in time to prevent harm. To be increasingly vigilant in an era of staffing shortages necessitates a strong defense against system failures, adequate training in complex technology, and sufficient information and coordination of team efforts in managing care.

Assessing and correlating data to identify potential, if not deadly, sentinel events began a century ago with a well-known nurse—Florence Nightingale. She was a risk reduction pioneer. She assessed the ghastly unsanitary conditions that were killing soldiers during the Crimean War, gathered data, and developed an action plan to improve care of the sick and wounded in the battlefield. She used her influence and persistence to make the necessary changes that would save countless lives. Her statistical charts describing the events (now displayed in the Florence Nightingale Museum in London) are some of the first epidemiological studies over time.

In this century, nurses have been filling out incident reports on errors since their student nurse days. These reports were countersigned and filed away, often leaving nurses feeling guilty and inadequate. It was not a positive learning experience, but one did develop a sense of responsibility that is part of the Code of Nursing. No other health care discipline was held to the same standard of incident reporting, and so nurses developed a sense of vigilance about their work that holds true today.

As chair of the Joint Commission's Accreditation Committee for the past four years, I have been part of the evolution of the Sentinel Event Policy, developed, in part, in response to the public reporting of sentinel event deaths in accredited health care organizations. Our committee was responsible for considering what actions to take, if any, concerning these events that were sensationalized to some degree in the media. Certainly, our committee raised many questions and discussed many issues. As a result of our deliberations, we developed a parallel investigative process to the usual survey and accreditation process and aimed to establish a level of confidentiality and security surrounding these sentinel events. Our goal was to learn from an intensive analysis of these sentinel events and to share the lessons learned with other health care organizations to prevent similar sentinel events.

Much has taken place since those initial discussions. The Accreditation Committee has reviewed and monitored over 1,100 sentinel events. We have moved from being judge and jury to students trying to understand the root causes that precipitated the event. People died, and you wondered how these events could occur. Our role was to determine if the organization had asked the relevant questions as to why it occurred. We encouraged organizations to seek the root causes and develop and implement an action plan to improve their systems.

Our committee also deemed it essential that we explore the role of the practitioners involved in the unanticipated death or serious complication—but not to levy punishment or blame. In the majority of cases reviewed, the practitioners were experienced professionals with positive performance evaluations in their files. They were not novices, nor were they temporary staff. They were nurses, doctors, pharmacists, and other health care professionals who were grieving because they had contributed in some way to a sentinel event that resulted in a death or serious adverse outcome. The prevailing culture depicted in the early root cause analysis of a sentinel event was predominantly one of blame—sentinel events were caused by human error. With considerable support from the Joint Commission staff and many educational programs and publications, the current root cause analysis suggests a new culture of systems review by team members with the focus on learning rather than blaming. This is a major turning point in promoting risk reduction throughout our health care systems. We need to analyze the facts, take corrective action, and share the learning with staff, not only with those involved, but also with staff throughout the organization. We aim to prevent such a situation from occurring again, rather than seeking out and blaming the individual and cloaking the event in secrecy and shame.

The case studies in this book are a composite of data that describe situations that can occur. Certainly, the case studies are compelling reading. You may question and wonder how these terrible events could have happened in a complex health care system with multiple checks and balances. That is exactly what this book wants you to do. That is how you will gain the insight and knowledge that will make you more vigilant in your nursing practice and in teaching future nurses. This valuable book offers many practical suggestions for assessing your organization's risk reduction strategies. As nurses on the front line 24 hours a day, seven days a week, your vigilance is what prevents "near misses" from turning into full-fledged sentinel events—but that is not enough. You need to determine how those "near misses" can be addressed and changes made so that the opportunity for a sentinel event to occur is minimized.

Unfortunately, despite our best efforts, errors will continue to be made in the health care system. However, we shouldn't give up. We need a multidisciplinary effort that focuses on the safety of our systems in health care organizations and the competence of our staff. This effort will make a difference in reducing the number of medical errors and sentinel events.

Nurses have been and always will be principal advocates for safe and compassionate care. The challenge for the nursing profession is to increase our vigilance in preventing sentinel events in a care delivery system where risks are inherent. We can't eliminate the risks completely, but through our vigilance, we can reduce them significantly. This book offers some helpful insights about risk reduction. Nurses—and, of course, all health care professionals—are also challenged by a serious nursing shortage, not only nationally but also globally. Given the complexity of our health care environment and the stress of understaffing, the potential for a sentinel event to occur is only magnified. All the more reason to learn from the lessons presented in this book.

Nurses play a major role in the mandate for health care safety because they should be encouraged to continue to seek solutions to protect the people in their care and the public. Nurses must use their influence as advocates for patient safety to promote a healing environment that constantly monitors its systems to minimize risks to individuals receiving care, families, and staff.

Sally Sample, RN, MN, FAAN
August 2001

Preface

Purpose of the Publication

Front Line of Defense: The Role of Nurses in Preventing Sentinel Events* is written for nurses working in all health care settings and specialties. Its goal is to further enhance a nurse's already formidable ability as advocate and caregiver to identify and prevent sentinel events in hospitals, ambulatory care, assisted living, behavioral health care, home care, and long term care organizations.

This publication includes examples of sentinel events from all types of health care organizations and prevention strategies applicable to all settings. How is this possible? Fundamental principles of nursing are applicable *wherever* nursing care is provided. Challenges or obstacles that must be addressed to prevent sentinel events, such as staffing, training, communication, and culture, are common to all health care organizations. Many of the studies reported in the health care literature and cited in this publication were conducted in acute care organizations. However, because of the universal role assumed by nurses and universal challenges to the safety of individuals receiving care, most of the lessons learned are applicable in all health care organizations.

Overview of Contents

Front Line of Defense: The Role of Nurses in Preventing Sentinel Events provides practical strategies nurses can use to identify and help prevent sentinel events. Because of the intended audience and goals of this publication, the strategies provided in this book focus on those related to the duties and responsibilities of nurses. This should not be interpreted as ignorance of the responsibilities of other members of the health care team. Nurses are not solely responsible for

protecting the health and safety of individuals in their care. However, in order to provide nurses with the most practical information, discussion in this book is limited to their particular role within the system.

Each chapter identifies a specific type of sentinel event that nurses have a potential to prevent, working as part of a team-oriented environment. Sentinel event categories were identified by Joint Commission staff and surveyors through the Joint Commission's Sentinel Event database and other nationally recognized studies on medical errors and health care safety. Because not all studies define sentinel event/error categories in the same way, readers may wish to consult the studies and reports identified in the *Resources* chapter for variations. A chapter-by-chapter description of this publication's contents follows.

The *Introduction* lays the groundwork for the publication, covering the nurse's role in contemporary health care; major challenges to safe care, including staffing issues, training, communication, and culture; and Joint Commission safety initiatives. Next, nine chapters address how nurses can take a leading role in change and help identify and prevent specific types of sentinel events: operative procedures and wrong-site surgeries (Chapter 1), medication errors (Chapter 2), transfusion errors (Chapter 3), injury or death resulting from falls (Chapter 4), infant abductions or releases to wrong families (Chapter 5), injury or death resulting from physical restraints (Chapter 6), elopements (Chapter 7), suicides (Chapter 8), and injury or death resulting from delays in treatment (Chapter 9). Each of the nine chapters includes an overview about why that particular sentinel event should be of concern to nurses and other health care team members, the major root causes of such events, and practical strategies nurses can use to reduce the likelihood of their occurrence.

Chapter 10 addresses nurses' roles in driving change to improve health care safety, and the role of education and continued competence in proactive health care safety efforts. The Appendix provides the full text of new and

---

* *Sentinel event*, as defined by the Joint Commission, is an unexpected occurrence involving death or serious physical or psychological injury, or the risk thereof. The term *sentinel* is used because these events sound a warning that requires immediate attention. A sentinel event involves an unexpected variation in a process or an outcome that demands notice, understanding, and action.

revised Joint Commission standards related to safety and error reduction. The Resources chapter guides readers to articles, books, and reports on the topic of sentinel events and error reduction, and an index enables readers to access topics by key word.

Confidentiality of Sentinel Event-Related Information

The Joint Commission vigorously protects the confidentiality of information learned during the accreditation process about sentinel events that occurred in health care organizations or the root cause analysis of such events. Hence, the examples of sentinel events included in chapters 1 through 9 of this publication do not describe any individual event occurring in any specific organization. The examples are composites and adaptations of incidents that have occurred in numerous organizations. No event has been presented as it actually occurred.

Use of this Publication

The strategies included in this publication illustrate ways that nurses in a variety of organizations have learned to identify the potential for sentinel events and reduce the likelihood of their occurrence. Some strategies may be applicable to your organization; some may not be. The key task for each reader is to use the strategies creatively and flexibly as a starting point for new or revised prevention systems, processes, and policies that are best suited to the organization's specific needs.

Publication of *Front Line of Defense: The Role of Nurses in Preventing Sentinel Events* does not in any way imply that nurses are to blame for sentinel events that do occur. Rather, the publication recognizes and celebrates nurses' unique, proactive opportunities to help identify and prevent systems-created errors. Whether or not nurses use the strategies outlined in this publication, individuals are not to blame for errors. Rather, errors result from faulty health care systems and processes.

A Note on Terminology

Throughout the publication, the words *individual receiving care* or *care recipient* are used to describe the person, client, consumer, patient, or resident who actually receives health care and services. Use of the word *patient* appears only when describing the individual receiving care in an acute care setting and when quoting material from health care literature.

Acknowledgments

Six Joint Commission surveyors invested many hours in providing examples and prevention strategies specific to each type of sentinel event. We wish to express our profound thanks to the following individuals for making this publication possible: Eddith Barrett, MS, RN, CS (Chapter 7); Joan Dodelin, BSN, MS (Chapter 5); Larry Grossman, MD (Chapters 1 and 3); Siward Hazelton, RN, MS (Chapters 8 and 9); Lynn A. Moran, RPh, BS, (Chapter 2); and Janet Sonnenberg, RN, MS, LNHA (Chapters 4 and 6). We also thank Nancy Haimen for organizing and writing this publication. We would like to extend special thanks to Sally A. Sample, RN, MN, FAAN for writing the Foreword for this book and for reviewing the manuscript.

Thanks as well to the following individuals who also reviewed this material: Diane Storer Brown, RN, PhD, CPHQ; Quality Outcomes Director, Kaiser Permanente; Mildred Delores Sawyer, RN, BSN, MPH; Surveyor, HEAST; Sam Fager, MD; Surveyor, ACAS; Anne Piper, RN; Surveyor, HCENT; Rita Munley Gallagher, PhD, RN, C, American Nurses Association; and Patricia Rowell, PhD, RN, Senior Policy Fellow, Department of Nursing Practice and Policy, American Nurses Association.

Introduction

Unique Roles in Contemporary Health Care

More than three million nursing personnel work in health care settings in the United States.[1] The term "nurse" embraces many different types of professionals including registered nurses (RNs), licensed practical nurses (LPNs), clinical nurse specialists, nurse practitioners, and nurse assistants (NAs). The size and scope of the roles played by nurses in hospitals, long term care facilities, assisted living facilities, behavioral health care organizations, ambulatory care facilities, and home care organizations cannot be overstated. Their roles are key. Minute-by-minute, hour-for-hour, and day-in and day-out, nurses provide a majority of the direct care received by individuals in all care settings. According to the American Hospital Association (AHA), nursing personnel provide 95% of the care an individual receives while hospitalized.[2] In all settings, nurses frequently are the first to observe improvements, changes, needs, and problems related to an individual's care and condition. They serve as frontline advocates for care recipients, communicating and coordinating with other health care professionals to help ensure that required adjustments to care plans and care provisions are made.

As such, nurses have a unique opportunity and responsibility to identify the potential for adverse or sentinel events related to individuals in their care and to prevent such events from occurring, where possible. Nurses do not function in a vacuum where their work is neither influenced by nor influences other staff and factors within the health care system. As such, like other health care professionals, they are *not* individually to blame for sentinel events. If a finger must be

pointed, faulty organizational systems and processes usually bear the blame. Organization leaders must ensure that nursing personnel are allowed to function as an integral part of a multi-disciplinary team and that the *whole* team is focused on improving health care processes and systems to reduce the likelihood of sentinel events and other adverse occurrences.

Trends in the health care industry have deeply impacted the settings in which nurses practice. As the bulk of care moved away from acute care settings during the past decades, nurses responded by meeting the need for care and services in home, ambulatory, behavioral health care, long term care, subacute care, and community-based health settings. Today, more nurses of all types are practicing in such settings rather than in the hospital setting. This reality shifts the focus of care interventions to include education, counseling, wellness and health maintenance, and integrated or continuing care delivery in home, community-based, and long term environments.[3]

Recent data from the nursing division of Health and Human Services' Health Resources and Services Administration illustrate the trend for the nation's 2.7 million active registered nurses. Of the active, licensed RNs in the United States, only 81.7% or 2.2 million are employed in nursing. This indicates that nurses are taking jobs in sectors beyond health care, thereby exacerbating nurse staffing shortages discussed later in this chapter. Whereas hospitals used to be the place of employment for the vast majority of RNs, only 59% of those employed in nursing remain in that setting, with 18% now working in public/community health, 10% in ambulatory

---

SIDEBAR I-1. OLD VERSUS NEW NURSING PARADIGMS

OLD PARADIGM	NEW PARADIGM
Success is based on high census.	Payer mix is more important than census.
Nurses are rewarded for working double shifts.	Nurses are rewarded for cognitive and critical thinking skills to achieve outcomes.
Full-time equivalent (FTE) staff counts are controlled to meet financial goals.	Cost per unit of service is controlled to meet goals.
Focus is on sick care and treatment.	Focus is on customer service.
Focus is on hospital care.	Focus is on caring for the individual in the right setting at the right time.

Source: Adapted from Beyers M (ed): *The Business of Nursing.* Chicago: American Hospital Publishing, 1996, p 12. Used with permission.

---

care, 7% in long term care, 2% in nursing education, and 4% in other settings.[4]

"The core of nursing service is threaded throughout the health care delivery system," writes Marjorie Beyers, PhD, RN, FAAN, then executive director of the American Organization of Nurse Executives (AONE).[5] Home care nurses may be the only agency professional seen by individuals receiving care at home. Nurses in the subacute and long term care setting are responsible for coordinating residents' care and usually hold primary responsibility for communicating with physicians and families. In ambulatory and behavioral health settings, nurses ensure coordinated medical care across the care continuum, often extending beyond the organizations' walls. Beyers advocates for the need to bring about changes in philosophy, attitude, and approach to nursing due to recent health care trends.[5] For example, nursing no longer focuses exclusively on acute care, but on providing care in the right setting at the right time. Shifts in thinking are mandatory as new paradigms take shape (see Sidebar I-1, above).

"Nurses go into the health care profession because they want to help people. Their patients' safety and well being is their primary concern and their sworn responsibility," writes Nancy Dickenson-Hazard, RN, MSN, CPNP, FAAN, executive officer of Sigma Theta Tau International the largest nursing honor society.[6] Indeed, the *Code for Nurses,* first adopted by the American Nurses Association (ANA) in 1950 and revised periodically throughout the years, addresses the nurse's advocacy role for those in their care and indicates that the nurse's primary commitment is to the health, welfare, and safety of the client. Code #3 reads, "The nurse acts to safeguard the client and the public when health care and safety are affected by the incompetent, unethical, or illegal practice of any person."[7] The interpretive statements outline the nurse's need to participate in the planning, establishment, implementation, and evaluation of review mechanisms that serve to safeguard clients. The ANA's *Standards of Clinical Nursing Practice* address the nurse's "safe, timely, and appropriate" implementation of interventions identified in the care plan; participation in quality of care activities; and evaluation of factors related to safety, effectiveness, availability, and cost when choosing between two or more practice options that would result in the same expected outcome.[8]

The quality of nursing care and nurses' ability to help protect the safety of those in their care are of vital importance to the public. In a public opinion poll conducted for the National Patient Safety Foundation (NPSF) by Louis Harris & Associates, 88% of consumers surveyed felt that nurses would have a positive effect on their safety as a health care recipient.[9] Nurses ranked third in individuals or groups likely to affect safety, following personal physicians and care recipients themselves. A Press, Ganey Associates satisfaction survey of one million past care recipients, conducted in the mid 1990s and cited by the ANA, indicated that six of the top 10 factors that affect likelihood to recommend a hospital relate to the quality of nursing care.[10] Both surveys indicate that the public believes that nurses have a positive effect on the safety and quality of care.

As front-line advocates for the individuals they serve, nurses are, in fact, the "sentinels" of care, sounding the warning for those in need of help and providing the help, as needed and feasible. Unfortunately, front-line players often suffer the bruises and other casualties resulting from high-stakes performance in an imperfect, highly-complex, and rapid-paced environment. High visibility and contact in the care arena makes nurses vulnerable to blame and punishment. Moreover, totem-pole ranking of health care professionals by discipline is still common in many organizations. Relegated to an inappropriate position at the bottom of the pole, nurses all too often are singled out as scapegoats.

Consider the continuing consequences for the nurses involved in the tragic and extensively publicized medication error that resulted in the death of a prominent reporter and one other woman at Boston's Dana-Farber Cancer Institute in 1994.[11] Following the incident, the Department of Public Health and the hospital itself conducted extensive investigations. Each concluded that the cause of the error was the failure of systems in place at the hospital, not of the individual nurses. The Joint Commission also conducted a survey of this organization. The hospital took full responsibility for the incident, publicly stating that the nurses should not be held accountable for the error. However, five years later, the Massachusetts Board of

Registration in Nursing announced its decision to pursue disciplinary sanctions against 16 of the 18 nurses involved. The two other nurses agreed with the board to have their licenses placed on probation for a year and to take continuing education in oncology nursing during that time. The state's board of medicine suspended the involved physician's right to renew his state license for three years, retroactive to 1995, and three pharmacists were reprimanded for their role in the error. Disciplinary action against the nurses, which can include revocation of licenses, is still pending as this book is published.

As noted in ANA's written testimony before a Senate committee on medical errors, "Despite increasing evidence that systems increasingly are failing to protect patients, the severity of discipline applied to providers for mistakes is increasing."[12] Consider the experience of the three nurses charged with criminally negligent homicide in an infant's death from a medication error in a Denver hospital in 1997. This case represented the first time that nurses faced criminal charges for making a medication error. The error involved the administration of a tenfold overdose of the intramuscular medication penicillin G benzathine by the intravenous route. The community was seeking individual accountability for what the prosecuting attorney described as a gross deviation from the standard of care that unjustifiably caused a risk to human health and safety.

With the threat of a conviction on homicide charges that would cost them their licenses for life and possibly result in jail terms, two of the nurses pleaded guilty. The third stood trial in January 1998. Staff of the Institute for Safe Medication Practices (ISMP) provided expert testimony and a systems analysis that identified more than 50 different "latent and active failures"[13] in the system that allowed the error to occur, remain undetected, and ultimately cause the death of a newborn child.[14] Recognizing that the error resulted from many system failures including unclear hospital policies and practices, inconsistent pharmacy procedures defining the prescriptive authority of non-physicians, and poor medication label design, the hospital supported the nurse by providing continued employment and legal defense funds. Later, the nurse was acquitted by a jury.

Thankfully, criminal prosecution for medical errors is not common practice. However, its emergence in the recent past attests to the tenacity of a culture of blame.

An Increasing Emphasis on Health Care Safety

Nurses and all types of health care professionals continue to step forward to meet the challenge of preventing health care errors. As one of the foremost challenges in the twenty-first century, safety of care recipients has gained increasing focus in the past five years. The reasons are three-fold.[15]

First, the evolution of, and revolution in, health care has had far-reaching consequences for the quality of care. As technological advances and delivery settings push health care into new frontiers, every type of health care organization is struggling with the need to provide more care and services with fewer resources. At the same time, the rapid explosion of biomedical and health knowledge has made it increasingly challenging for practitioners to stay current. In general, workloads have become heavier, creating increased stress and fatigue for health care professionals. Caregivers are working in new settings and performing new functions, sometimes with minimal training. Skill mixes are shifting. These and other factors have exacerbated the opportunity for serious medical errors.

Second, public awareness of, and concern about, health care safety has increased dramatically. As mentioned earlier, a number of nationally publicized adverse events in 1994 and 1995 triggered issues of public trust in health care. Some of these events occurred in health care organizations that have long-standing, excellent reputations. Consulting with experts within health care and other high-risk endeavors (for example, airline and nuclear power industries), the Joint Commission developed its Sentinel Event Policy. Implemented nationally for all Joint Commission-accredited organizations in

1996, this policy emphasizes the identification, analysis, and sharing of sentinel event-related information. Detailed information on the policy appears in Joint Commission accreditation manuals, publications, and Web site (*www.jcaho.org*).

Third, the impetus to address errors, pioneered by such figures as Florence Nightingale and Ernest A. Codman, was reinvigorated in the mid 1990s. At that time, the Joint Commission partnered with other opinion leaders and expert organizations to highlight the need for action on safety within health care. A groundbreaking international expert conference was co-convened in 1996 by the Joint Commission with the American Association for the Advancement of Science, the American Medical Association, and the Annenberg Center for Health Sciences at Eisenhower Medical Center, and co-sponsored by eleven other agencies, including the then-Agency for Health Care Policy and Research, associations, foundations, and industry representatives. Titled *Examining Errors in Health Care: Developing a Prevention, Education, and Research Agenda,* this multidisciplinary conference was an important starting point in the development of an agenda for making error reduction a common goal. Many stakeholders in the health care safety arena launched their initiatives at or following this conference or its sequel events.

Released in November 1999, the Institute of Medicine's (IOM) report, *To Err is Human: Building a Safer Health System,* catalyzed the professional and policy-making communities and public at large around the critical issue of health care safety.[16] Public awareness of, and concern about, health care safety now appears to have reached an all-time high. According to a survey released in December 2000 by the Kaiser Family Foundation and the Agency for Healthcare Research and Quality (AHRQ), 47% of adults surveyed expressed serious doubts about obtaining error-free services in health care in general, and specifically in hospitals.[17] This percentage is five points higher than data from a public opinion poll cited earlier, which found that 42% of adults surveyed believed that the current health care system does not have adequate measures in place to prevent medical mistakes.[9] Individuals may always have felt some trepidation about the possibility of falling victim to medical error. However, with the release of the IOM report, it seemed that overnight the public shifted from viewing incidents as unlikely anomalies to fearing that they are commonplace. This highlights perhaps the costliest aspect of medical error—the loss of trust in the health care system.

On March 1, 2001, the IOM released its second and final report, *Crossing the Quality Chasm: A New Health System for the 21st Century.*[18] The report describes the U.S. health care system as "a tangled, highly fragmented web that often leaves unaccountable gaps in care and fails to build on the strengths of all health professionals."[19] It calls for immediate action to improve care and offers a comprehensive strategy to do so. Part of that strategy is monitoring and tracking by the U.S. Department of Health and Human Services of quality improvements in six key areas: safety, effectiveness, responsiveness of patients, timeliness, efficiency, and equity. According to the report, safety will be achieved not by asking health care workers to work harder, but by fundamentally changing the way in which care is organized and delivered.

Moving Away From a Blameful Society

As mentioned earlier, the desire to assign individual blame for errors is all too prevalent in contemporary society. Perhaps it emanates from the destructive need to root out the culprit by seeking an eye for an eye. The myth of perfect performance creates feelings of emotional distress and inadequacy from anyone making a mistake. If that mistake occurs in the health care arena where the Hippocratic Oath's "First do no harm" is so firmly ingrained, and if the health care professional's mistake causes harm, guilt and remorse predominate. The perpetrator becomes "the culprit" or "the bad apple" to be rooted out.

The pressure to be perfect provides strong incentive to cover up mistakes rather than to

disclose them and address underlying root causes.* So do recent sensationalist headlines, such as those from the *Chicago Tribune* exclaiming, "Nursing mistakes kill, injure thousands," "Nursing accidents unleash silent killer," and "Problem nurses escape punishment."[20] These headlines add fuel to the fire. All too often, nurses see jobs lost and licenses revoked when blame is assigned to nurse colleagues. It is no wonder then that they may fear reporting sentinel events or the potential for such events.

Responding to the *Chicago Tribune* articles, Ann O'Sullivan, RN, president of the Illinois Nurses Association, writes, "The fact is nurses are a patient's best safety net in the hospital. Every day nurses prevent countless problems and complications, catch mistakes before they happen, and try to provide the very best care possible in extremely difficult situations. When that safety net gets stretched too thin, mistakes are more likely to happen. . ."[21] In fact, if one reads beyond the headlines of the *Tribune* articles, the author identifies appropriate systems-oriented causes for errors, including inadequate staffing and insufficient training.

The blame and punishment orientation of society drives errors underground. A poll conducted by Peter D. Hart Research Associates in the mid 1990s found that one-fourth of health care professionals were afraid to speak up about problems they saw in their daily work.[22] A new study, which surveyed medical and nursing staff working in U.S. intensive care units, found that many errors are neither acknowledged nor discussed by health care staff because of personal reputation (76%), the threat of malpractice suits (71%), possible disciplinary actions by licensing boards (64%), and threat to job security (63%).[23] The authors conclude that substantial pressures still exist to cover up mistakes, thereby overlooking opportunities for improvement.

New Joint Commission safety and health care error reduction standards[†] address the need for leaders to develop a culture that emphasizes cooperation and communication in order to improve safety. Communication must

---

* An in-depth discussion of root causes, including how to conduct a root cause analysis, can be found in *Root Cause Analysis In Health Care: Tools and Techniques,* published by Joint Commission Resources in 2000.

[†] These standards as approved for use in hospitals appear in the Appendix at the back of the book.

include information about potential and actual sentinel events. Legislation providing protection to health care workers who speak out about problems in their organizations also aims to alleviate the pressure to cover up mistakes. To date the following states have whistleblower protection laws: Oregon, West Virginia, California, Kentucky, Massachusetts, Minnesota, New Jersey, Texas, and Wisconsin. As of publication, similar laws have been introduced in Hawaii, Illinois, Missouri, New York, Oregon, Pennsylvania and Rhode Island. This legislation generally protects nurses and other health care professionals from retaliation by their employers if they "blow the whistle" on hazardous practices that jeopardize an individual's safety.[24] Retaliation includes, for example, disciplinary action and the threat of disciplinary action, for initiating, participating, or testifying about a violation of state or federal laws or regulations. Nurses and other health care professionals are also protected for blowing the whistle when the quality of any health care service provided by an organization or an employee violates standards established by state or federal law or regulation.[24] Similarly, they are protected when the service violates clinical or ethical standards established by a professionally recognized accrediting or standard-setting body and poses a potential risk to public health or safety.[24]

Experts and organizations at the forefront of efforts to reduce medical errors recognize errors as the symptoms of systems diseases. The diseases, not the symptoms, must be treated. Blaming an individual does not change the factors contributing to the error. The error is likely to recur. For example, one organization treated the *symptom* of a medication error by firing the nurse who administered the wrong medication. Another organization treated the *disease* itself by developing and implementing a new labeling system to prevent the recurrence of the medication error. Lasting change that reduces the future probability of errors is brought about only through systems improvement.*

The key systems issues most frequently cited to be at the root of sentinel events involve staffing, training, communication, and culture. These represent the greatest challenge to the provision of safe care by all health care professionals.

Staffing and Training

Proper staffing helps to ensure the safety of those receiving care and treatment. The correlation between effective staffing and positive health care outcomes is highly studied. Some studies in the literature cite a direct link between appropriate nurse staffing levels, staff mix, quality care, and health care outcomes. The debate about nurse staffing levels and mix is highly charged in contemporary health care.

The Joint Commission supports a broad approach to the issue of staffing adequacy. No specific ratios of nursing or other organizational staff to individuals are prescribed. Rather, the Joint Commission is concerned that an organization must have an adequate supply of staff to meet the needs of individuals receiving care. Through its Management of Human Resources, Improving Organizational Performance, and Leadership standards that appear in all accreditation manuals, the Joint Commission provides health care organizations seeking and maintaining accreditation with a systematic approach to address staffing needs. Leaders must define staff qualifications and performance expectations; provide adequate numbers of competent staff; orient, train, and educate that staff; and assess competence on an ongoing basis. Organizations are required to ensure that the needs of both the organization and the individuals in its care drive the mix of required staff qualifications.

New standards addressing staffing effectiveness have been approved for implementation in hospitals in July 2002.[†] Implementation of comparable standards for other Joint Commission accreditation programs is being considered.

In today's health care environment, discussions of staff-to-care recipient ratios abound. An IOM

---

* Although a full discussion of how and why errors occur and the proactive design of error-proof health care processes is beyond this book's scope, readers may wish to consult other books and articles in the *Resources* chapter.

---

† As of this publication, these standards are available for viewing at the Joint Commission Web site at *www.jcaho.org.*

report on nursing staff adequacy in hospitals and nursing homes[1] concluded that there was no solid evidence of a decline in the quality of hospital care because of any changes in staffing. The committee issuing the report rejected the idea of mandatory minimum nurse staffing levels in hospitals, and concluded that "there is a serious paucity of recent research on the definitive effects of structural measures, such as specific staffing ratios, on the quality of patient care in terms of patient outcomes when controlling for all other likely explanatory or confounding variables."[25] For example, improved mortality indicators in hospitals with RN-rich staffing ratios cited in one study[26] were "likely due to other attributes of hospitals that grant nurses autonomy over their own practice and control of the resources necessary to deliver patient care and create good relationships with physicians. . . The issue is not just a matter of staffing ratios. . . what RNs do and how they do it are both more important than simply how many RNs there are," note the report authors.[25]

The AHA opposes mandated nurse staffing ratios. "Nurse staffing should be driven by patient needs, and hospitals need flexibility to make sure they can put qualified caregivers in the right place at the right time to meet patient needs. A rigid, one-size-fits-all approach to staffing does a disservice to patients and nurses alike by failing to account for patient acuity and nurse experience," notes that organization.[27] One state hospital association states that, "Although high nurse-patient ratios are intuitively appealing, legislating a bright line in this area may not serve patient safety objectives and may impair the ability of hospitals to provide timely access to hospital care."[28] The organizations' recommendations include focusing on the larger problem of the work force, specifically nursing shortages, and developing long-term national strategies to attract and retain young people in the nursing field.

Nursing organizations are more likely to represent a different view. In May 2000, the ANA released the results of a study that quantifies nursing's impact on health care outcomes.[29] The study, which augmented earlier ANA studies,[30,31] is part of ANA's Safety and Quality Initiative, a multi-phased effort to promote the use of

objective measures to demonstrate relationships between nurse staffing and outcomes. Using hospital and Medicare data from nine states, the study looked at outcome measures involving morbidities "that can. . . be theorized to be preventable in some individuals by the amount and skill mix of nursing care provided."[29] Measures included length of stay, postoperative infections, pressure ulcers, and urinary tract infections. Each of the outcome measures showed statistically significant correlations with nurse staffing. Shorter lengths of stay were related to higher levels of overall nurse staffing. Lower than expected complication rates were associated with a higher mix of RNs among licensed nursing personnel for all four adverse complications. "Not only do patients do better, but hospitals can actually save money by using highly skilled nurses in adequate numbers," writes ANA president, Mary Foley, MS, RN.[32]

On the national level, the Code of Federal Regulations' Conditions of Participation for Hospitals (42 CFR 82) addresses nurse staffing only in the hospital setting and only for hospitals receiving Medicare and Medicaid payments. It states, "The nursing service must have adequate numbers of licensed registered nurses, licensed practical (vocational) nurses, and other personnel to provide nursing care to all patients as needed."[33] This code is under review.

Given the lack of a more prescriptive national standard, a number of state legislatures have stepped in to begin establishing staffing requirements in such settings as critical care units and operating rooms. California is the furthest along in the process at this point. In October 1999, its governor signed the California Patient Safety Act, establishing requirements for nurse-to-patient ratios by licensed nurse classification and hospital unit. The California Nurses Association and the ANA have not developed specific numeric ratios, believing that a broader approach to nurse staffing in acute care settings is needed, one supplemented by an accurate and reliable acuity/patient classification system.[34] Since the fall of 1999, approximately 21 states have introduced legislation related to staffing issues, the bulk of which have been spearheaded by nursing organizations.[28]

In the long term care setting, the issue of minimum nurse staffing has been debated since the Omnibus Budget Reconciliation Act of 1987 (OBRA 87). Following passage of OBRA 87, the Centers for Medicare and Medicaid Services (CMS) (formerly the Health Care Financing Administration or HCFA) issued regulations that included a general requirement that nursing homes must provide

> ". . . a sufficient nursing staff to attain or maintain the highest practicable. . . well-being of each resident. . ."

In studying the relationship between nurse staffing and quality of care, the IOM's Committee on the Adequacy of Nurse Staffing in Hospitals and Nursing Homes concluded that, "The preponderance of evidence from a number of studies using different types of quality measures has shown a positive relationship between nursing staff levels and quality of nursing home care, indicating a strong need to increase the overall level of nursing staff in nursing homes."[35] The committee recommended increasing levels of all nursing staff (RNs, LPNs, and NAs) in long term care facilities, and increasing RN coverage in all facilities on all shifts. However, the committee indicated that prescribing a staffing ratio across all residents and facilities was an inadequate approach due to "varying circumstances among nursing homes and case-mix differential within and between facilities."[36]

Public and congressional concern about nurse staffing in long term care organizations was heightened by the CMS's nursing home report to Congress in 1998 that identified a range of serious safety and quality of care problems, including malnutrition, dehydration, pressure sores, abuse, and neglect. State licensure agencies responded by imposing new, more stringent staffing requirements. The majority of states—37—have some type of nurse staffing requirements for nursing homes, but the requirements vary considerably.[36] Twenty-eight states specify the required hours of nursing care per resident day; eleven states specify a staff member-to-resident ratio; and seven states outline the required number of registered nursing hours.

In August 2000, the CMS released Phase 1 of a new report to Congress, titled *Appropriateness of Minimum Nurse Staffing Ratios in Nursing Homes*.[36] The report's review of prior research on the relationship between staffing and resident outcomes revealed no consistently strong positive or negative association. However, the report also summarized results of an empirical study of the relationship between staffing and quality. The study examined both positive outcomes, such as improvements in activities of daily living functioning and resident cleanliness and grooming, and negative outcomes, such as avoidable hospitalizations, incidence of pressure sores, and weight loss. Time-motion studies defined the minimal staffing necessary to provide optimal care in delivering five specific daily care services. "Strong associations between low staffing and the likelihood of quality problems across these measures, adjusted for risks were found for all nurse staffing," states the report.[36]

With continually shrinking reimbursement and shortages of trained and experienced personnel, all health care organizations are struggling to define and attain an optimum level and mix of nurses that ensures the provision of quality care. Estimates on nursing vacancies are alarming, with experts predicting shortages of 100,000 to 500,000 nurses by 2020.[4] A steady decline in nursing school enrollment, the aging of the current nurse population, and increased demand for nursing services as the U.S. population grows and ages make it likely that the struggle will continue well into the future.

Trends related to staffing adequacy, such as mandatory overtime, "speed-up" through increased workloads, and the use of unlicensed staff to perform duties normally assumed in the licensed nursing domain, are cited frequently in health care literature as error-prone staffing strategies. "(Speeding up). . . means that nurses are expected to work harder and faster with fewer resources, providing care for greater numbers of sicker people in the same amount of time. Such a pattern invariably leads to a higher turnover and an increase in work-related injuries, and ultimately jeopardizes quality of care," notes one source.[37]

The professional literature includes accounts of the increased risk of error and harm to recipients of care due to the increased use of unlicensed and untrained staff. Insufficient training certainly increases the potential for error. Lucien Leape, MD, MPH, a leading advocate of systems-based approaches to reducing health care error, said that "decreasing the expertise of (health care) personnel by replacing highly skilled nurses with lesser trained people. . . [is leading to the creation of] accidents waiting to happen."[38]

Training and continuing education frequently suffer during staffing shortages. Most health care organizations regularly experience the challenge of finding time for staff training. Who will cover while a nurse is attending a continuing education or training session? Training time frames for registered nurses have been shortened and cross-training is common. Veteran nurses are hard-pressed to find any space or time to mentor less experienced nurses. They are simply too busy with direct care provision. "Floating" nurses are asked to assume wider responsibilities, and many RNs are required to work in care areas where they believe they have scanty orientation, training, experience, or support.[34]

In order to reduce the likelihood of adverse events, nurses need to be able to spend an appropriate amount of time with individuals in their care. Technological advances enabling complex medical and nursing procedures combined with increased acuity of care needs create an environment ripe for error. Nurses are those individuals who are watching the monitors, reading the gauges, recording the data, and managing the increasingly sophisticated technological devices to "keep them ticking, timing, and ever engaged," write two experts.[39] Not surprisingly, a recent survey conducted by the ANA found that 56% of the 7,300 RNs surveyed believed that the time they have available for direct care has decreased.[40]

Communication and Culture

Nurses provide continuity of care for individuals in all health care settings. Observing the individual on a regular basis, they can identify changes in condition or behavior indicating

problems or the need for care plan revision. In most settings, the opportunity for error increases as the number of staff involved in one individual's care rises. Coordination of care among health care professionals through an interdisciplinary care-management process and coordinated communication are vital to safety. Yet all too often, organization leaders need to make interdisciplinary collaboration more of a priority. Hierarchical "pecking orders" interfere with properly coordinated care focused on meeting the individual's needs.

Reduced staffing heightens the critical need for a multidisciplinary approach to error reduction. Writes one author: "Reduced staffing has forced us to acknowledge professional interdependence and the need for collaboration among physicians, pharmacists, nurses, and patients."[41] The ISMP urges "work(ing) together, side by side, to create safety for the system as a whole, rather than within single disciplines, departments, or units," and "new strategies or novel combinations of safety measures that have been previously performed only within each profession."[42] For example, a multidisciplinary team is key to medication error reduction efforts. Physician-pharmacist-nurse collaboration and improvements in automation, such as bar code systems, can help reduce medication errors.

Health care organizations must ensure an environment and culture conducive to communication and collaboration. A hierarchical culture can make nurses reluctant to raise concerns or question physicians and pharmacists about medications, dosages, and other elements of care. In its February 2000 report to the president, the Quality Interagency Coordination Task Force wrote,

> Because of the nature of medical errors, an effective response requires an integration of efforts across traditional occupational and scientific boundaries. The nature of the patient safety challenge requires synergy among scientific and technical disciplines, from human factors psychology to product design and delivery. This collaboration is needed at all stages of the effort to reduce errors and enhance patient safety—from research on its causes and remedies to implementation and partnership in its

reduction and elimination. The response to medical errors by the health care system is hindered by the traditional focus of single disciplines on individual providers or on products. . . [43]

To make this happen, a new health care culture often is needed. "Despite the many adjectives (interdisciplinary, multidisciplinary, transprofessional, interprofessional) used to describe this approach in the new health care culture, the concept remains constant—health professionals from different disciplines working together to provide a continuum of preventive and health care services to address the needs of patients whose continuum of care extends beyond hospital walls," says one author.[44] The new models of collaboration cannot be hierarchical: rather, they must be team oriented.

Joint Commission Initiatives

The safety of health care has been an integral part of the Joint Commission's mission since the organization's inception. The Joint Commission has developed state of the art, professionally based standards and evaluated the compliance of health care organizations against these benchmarks since 1951. An analysis of current standards indicates that nearly 50% of Joint Commission accreditation requirements relate to issues of health care safety. As Joint Commission president Dennis S. O'Leary, MD, notes, this link is due to the fact that

> . . . the accreditation process is, at its core, a risk reduction activity. It begins with the setting of contemporary standards that address important organization functions—for example, patient assessment, medication usage—and then encourages organizations, through the awarding of accreditation, to comply with these standards. The operating thesis is that if organizations are doing the 'right things right,' as reflected in the standards, then errors and adverse outcomes are less likely to happen than if there were no such standards. Notwithstanding the continued high frequency of errors, this thesis is almost certainly correct.[45]

The Joint Commission holds that information is at the core of health care error reduction

efforts. In testimony before House and Senate committees in February 2000, O'Leary outlined the following five critical, information-based tasks whose completion is essential to an effective error-reduction strategy:[46]

1. Create a blame-free, protected environment that encourages the systematic surfacing and reporting of serious adverse events;

2. Produce credible "root cause" analyses of serious adverse events;

3. Implement concrete, planned actions to reduce the likelihood of similar errors in the future;

4. Establish safety standards which health care organizations must meet; and

5. Disseminate experiential information learned from errors to all organizations at risk for serious adverse events.

The Joint Commission addresses each of these tasks through its Sentinel Event Policy and program, and safety and health care error reduction standards. A detailed description of the Sentinel Event Policy can be found in accreditation manuals and on the Joint Commission's Web site (*www.jcaho.org*). Statistics on sentinel events reviewed by the Joint Commission since 1995 as part of the policy's mission appear as Table I-1, page xvii. The number of reported errors represents only the tip of the iceberg. The most common root causes of sentinel events reported to the Joint Commission appear in Figure I-1, page xviii.

In 1997, the Joint Commission began to issue periodic *Sentinel Event Alerts* to share the most important lessons learned from its database of sentinel events-known risks in systems and processes as well as safe practices. Newsletter issues appear in Sidebar I-2, page XX.

Safety and Health Care Error Reduction Standards

The second major Joint Commission safety initiative affecting nurses and other health care professionals was the incorporation of appropriate information learned from the analysis of sentinel events into accreditation standards.

Table I-1. Sentinel Event Statistics

Total Number of Sentinel Events Reviewed by the Joint Commission Since January 1995	1,398

Type of Sentinel Event	#	%
Patient suicide	242	17.3%
Op/post-op complication	168	12.0%
Medication error	162	11.6%
Wrong-site surgery	148	10.6%
Delay in treatment	73	5.2%
Pt. death/injury in restraints	69	4.9%
Patient fall	67	4.8%
Assault/rape/homicide	60	4.3%
Patient elopement	31	2.2%
Perinatal death/loss of function	36	2.6%
Transfusion error	35	2.5%
Fire	29	2.1%
Infant abduction/wrong family	23	1.6%
Anesthesia-related event	20	1.4%
Med equipment-related	19	1.4%
Ventilator death/injury	23	1.6%
Maternal death	18	1.3%
Death assoc. w/transfer	14	1.0%
Other less frequent types	161	11.5%

Settings of Sentinel Events	#	%
General hospital	869	62.2%
Psychiatric hospital	194	13.9%
Psych unit in general hospital	93	6.7%
Behavioral health facility	77	5.5%
Long term care facility	57	4.1%
Emergency department	53	3.8%
Home care	31	2.2%
Ambulatory care	19	1.4%
Clinical laboratory	4	0.3%
Health care network	1	0.1%

Sources for SE Identification	#	%
Self-report	952	68.1%
Media	189	13.5%
Complaints	123	8.8%
Identified during survey	85	6.6%
Other (e.g., CMS report)	43	3.1%

Sentinel Event Outcomes	#	%
Patient death	1105	75%
Loss of Function	133	9%
Other	231	16%
Total patients impacted	1469	100%

Legend: *Since 1995, the Joint Commission has reviewed approximately 1,400 sentinel events. This table provides information on the types of sentinel events reviewed, their settings, sources for sentinel event identification, and sentinel event outcomes as of August 30, 2001.*

The Joint Commission-approved standards directly focus on the safety of those receiving care and medical/health care error reduction. Implemented for hospitals effective July 2001, the initiative will extend to other programs over time. The standards are designed to improve health care safety and reduce risk to care recipients. They go beyond retrospective analysis of events to focus on proactively creating a culture of safety in health care organizations. They emphasize the proactive safety engineering of health care processes—using such techniques as failure mode, effects, and criticality analysis—safety education of staff, and disclosure to the care recipient and family of significant unanticipated outcomes in care.

Although the standards focus on the safety of those receiving care, an organization-wide safety initiative also includes staff (nurses and other health care professionals) and visitors. Many of the activities taken to improve health care safety (for example, security, equipment safety, infection control) encompass staff and visitors as well as care recipients.

Effective reduction of medical/health care errors and other factors that contribute to unintended adverse health care outcomes in a health care organization requires an environment in which care recipients, their families, nurses, and other organization staff and leaders can identify and manage actual and potential risks to safety. This environment encourages

■ recognition and acknowledgment of risks to care recipient safety and medical/health care errors;

■ the initiation of actions to reduce these risks; the internal reporting of what has been found and the actions taken;

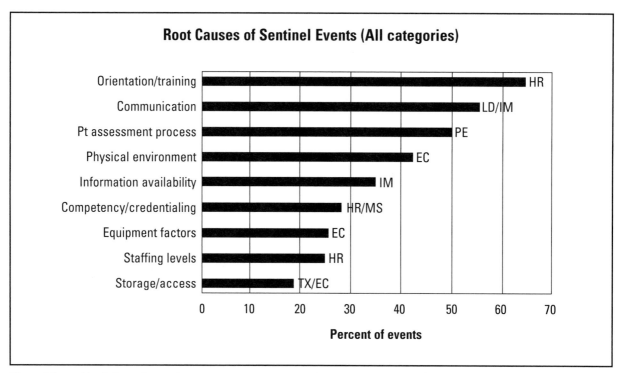

Figure I-1. *provides information on the most common root causes identified for sentinel events reviewed by the Joint Commission. Organizations completing a root cause analysis of a sentinel event in their facility identified insufficient orientation/training and communication problems as root causes of approximately 55 to 65 percent of reviewed events.*

SIDEBAR I-2. *SENTINEL EVENT ALERT:* NEWSLETTER ISSUES*

Blood Transfusion Errors: Preventing Future Occurrences

Fatal Falls: Lessons for the Future

Exposure to Creutzfeldt-Jakob Disease

High-Alert Medications and Patient Safety

Infant Abductions: Preventing Future Occurrences

Infusion Pumps: Preventing Future Adverse Events

Inpatient Suicides: Recommendations for Prevention

Kernicterus Threatens Healthy Newborns

Lessons Learned: Wrong Site Surgery

Lessons Learned: Fires in the Home Care Setting

Look-alike, Sound-alike Drug Names

Mix-up Leads to a Medication Error

Medication Error Prevention—Potassium Chloride

Operative and Post-Operative Complications: Lessons for the Future

Preventing Restraint Deaths

Medical Gas Mixups

Preventing Needlestick and Sharps Injuries

Legend: *Full newsletter issues may be accessed on the Joint Commission's Web site:* www.jcaho.org.

* List complete as of publication date

■ a focus on processes and systems; and minimization of individual blame or retribution for involvement in a medical/health care error; and

■ organizational learning about medical/health care errors and sharing of that knowledge to effect behavioral changes in itself and other health care organizations to improve the safety of those receiving care.

The full text of the Safety and Health Care Error Reduction standards for hospitals appears in the Appendix, pages 129–144. Implementation of comparable standards for other Joint Commission accreditation programs is anticipated in 2002 to 2003.

Concluding Comments

As front-line providers of direct care in all health care settings, nurses are key to the success of many strategies aimed at identifying and preventing sentinel events. In their unique role as health care team members, nurses can have a critical impact on the safety of those in their care. Nine chapters outlining proactive strategies nurses can use to reduce the likelihood of sentinel events follow. A full description of each chapter's contents appears in the Preface (pages vii–viii). Even though the strategies provided here are tailored for nurses, the reader must appreciate the fact that nurses do not and cannot work in a vacuum, nor are they or any other type of professional individually responsible for health care errors. Health care organization leaders must ensure multidisciplinary teamwork and ensure that the whole team is focused on improving faulty processes and systems to improve health care safety.

References

1. Wunderlich GD, Sloan FA, Davis CK: *Nursing Staff in Hospitals and Nursing Homes: Is It Adequate?* Report from the Institute of Medicine's Committee on the Adequacy of Nurse Staffing in Hospitals and Nursing Homes. Washington, DC: National Academy Press, 1996, p. 69.

2. American Hospital Association: *Hospital Nurse Recruitment and Retention, A Source Book for Executive Management.* No date. Chicago, IL: American Hospital Association.

3. Beyers M (Ed): *The Business of Nursing.* Chicago, IL: American Hospital Publishing, 1996, p. 61.

4. Health Resources and Services Administration (HHS): *2000 National Sample Survey of Registered Nurses.* Washington, DC: HRSA, 2000.

5. Beyers M (1996), *Opcit,* pps. ix–xi.

6. Sigma Theta Tau International, Nursing Honor Society: Dickenson-Hazard responds to *Chicago Tribune* articles. Sep 15, 2000. Web site: *www.nursingsociety.org.*

7. American Nurses Association: *Code for Nurses with Interpretive Statements.* Washington, DC: American Nurses Association, 1985.

8. American Nurses Association: *Standards of Clinical Nursing Practice: 2nd Edition.* Washington, DC: American Nurses Publishing, 1998.

9. National Patient Safety Foundation at the American Medical Association: *Public Opinion of Patient Safety Issues: Research Findings.* Sep 1997. Web site: *www.npsf.org.*

10. As cited in American Nurses Association: Consumers' concerns about health care echo nurses' warnings says ANA. Press release, Jan 31, 1997. Web site: *www.nursingworld.org/pressrel/1997/surveys.htm.*

11. Trossman S: ANA, MNA support Dana-Farber nurses facing disciplinary action. *MassNurs News,* Apr/May 1999. Web site: *www.massnurses.org.*

12. Foley M: Written testimony of the American Nurses Association before the Senate Committee on Health, Education, Labor and Pensions on Medical Errors, Jan 26, 2000. Web site: *www.nursingworld.org/gova/federal/legis/testimon/2000/mf0126htm.*

13. Reason J: *Human Error.* Cambridge University Press, 1990.

14. Institute for Safe Medication Practices: Lessons from Denver: look beyond blaming individuals for errors. *ISMP Medication Safety Alert!* Feb 11, 1998. Web site: *www.ismp.org/MSAarticles/Denver.html.*

15. Schyve PM: Statement of the Joint Commission on Accreditation of Healthcare Organizations at the National Summit of Medical Errors and Patient Safety Research. Sep 11, 2000. Web site: *www.jcaho.org/sentinel/se_summit.html.*

16. Institute of Medicine report: *To err is human: Building a safer health system.* Washington, DC: National Academy Press, 2000.

17. Kaiser Family Foundation and the Agency for Healthcare Research and Quality: *National Survey on Americans as Health Care Consumers: An Update on the Role of Quality Information.* Dec 2000. Web site: *www.kff.org.*

18. Institute of Medicine report: *Crossing the Quality Chasm: A New Health System for the 21st Century.* Washington, DC: National Academy Press, 2001.

19. National Academy Press Release: U.S. health care delivery system needs major overhaul to improve quality and safety. March 1, 2001. Web site: *www4. nationalacademies.org/news.nsf/isbn/0309072808? OpenDocument.*

20. A three-part series by Michael J. Berens published by the *Chicago Tribune* on Sep 10–12, 2000.

21. O'Sullivan A: Patient advocates (editorial). *Chicago Tribune*, Sep 17, 2000.

22. As cited in Comment & Opinion: Protecting the patient by protecting the worker. *Amer Nurse.* Sep/Oct 1998. Web site: *www.nursingworld.org/tan/ 98sepoct/protect.htm.*

23. Sexton JB, Thomas EJ, Helreich RL: Error, stress, and teamwork in medicine and aviation: Cross sectional surveys. *BMJ* 320:745–749, 18 Mar 2000.

24. Elliott SJ: Health care whistleblower legislation. *Health Law Alert,* Mar 2000. Milwaukee, WS: vonBriesen, Purtell & Roper. Web site: *www. vonbriesen.com/whistleblower.htm.*

25. Wunderlich et al (1996), *Opcit,* pp. 121–122.

26. Aiken LH, Smith HL, Lake ET: Lower Medicare mortality among a set of hospitals known for good nursing care. *Medical Care* 32(8):771–787, 1994.

27. American Hospital Association: Improving patient care and reducing the regulatory burden. Web site: *www.aha.org.*

28. Illinois Hospital & Healthsystems Association: Position paper on nursing staffing. Jan 18, 2001. Web site: *www.ihha.org.*

29. American Nurses Association: *Nurse Staffing and Patient Outcomes in the Inpatient Hospital Setting.* Washington, DC: American Nurses Publishing, 2000.

30. American Nurses Association: *Nursing Care Report Card for Acute Care.* Washington, DC: American Nurses Association, 1995.

31. Knauf RA, Lichtig LK, Rison-McCoy AD, et al: *Implementing Nursing's Report Card: A Study of RN Staffing, Length of Stay and Patient Outcomes.* Washington, DC: American Nurses Association, 1997.

32. ANA Press Release: New ANA study provides more proof of link between RN staffing and quality patient care. Washington, DC: American Nurses Association, May 2, 2000. Web site: *www.nursing-world.org/rnrealnews.*

33. *House of Delegates Action Report, ANA House of Delegates.* Washington, DC: American Nurses Association, 2000.

34. Romig CL: Health policy issues: Developing a nurse-to-patient ratio policy. *AORN Journal,* Nov 2000. Web site: *www.aorn.org/ journal/nov2khpi.htm.*

35. Wunderlich et al (1996), *Opcit,* p. 153.

36. Appropriateness of Minimum Nurse Staffing Ratios in Nursing Homes. HCFA Report to Congress, Aug 1, 2000. Web site: *www.hcfa.gov/medicaid/reports/ rp700hmp.htm.*

37. ANA Press Release: Consumers' concerns about health care echo nurses' warnings says ANA. Jan 31, 1997. Web site: *www.nursingworld.org/ pressrel/1997/surveys.htm.*

38. Leape LL: Address to National Patient Safety Foundation news conference, Chicago, IL, Oct 7, 1997.

39. Weaver DJ, Rimar JM: Understanding the patient care executive's changing role and responsibilities. In Beyers M (Ed): *The Business of Nursing.* Chicago, IL: American Hospital Publishing, 1996, p. 2.

40. Gardner J: Survey: Nurses feeling overworked. *Modern Healthcare,* Feb 23, 2001, p. 12.

41. Knox GE et al: Downsizing, reengineering and patient safety: numbers, new-ness and resultant risk. *J Health Risk Manag* 1999; 19:18–25.

42. ISMP: Maintaining patient safety in the face of staff reduction. *ISMP Medication Safety Alert,* Oct 20, 1999. Web site: *www.ismp.org/MSAarticles/ staffing.html.*

43. Quality Interagency Coordination Task Force: *Doing what counts for patient safety: Federal actions to reduce medical errors and their impact.* Report to the President, Feb 2000.

44. Felton G: Facing nursing's new educational challenges. In Beyers M (Ed): *The Business of Nursing.* Chicago, IL: American Hospital Publishing, 1996, pp. 69–78.

45. O'Leary DS: Editorial: Accreditation's role in reducing medical errors. *BMJ* 320:727–8, Mar 2000.

46. O'Leary D: Statement of the Joint Commission on Accreditation of Healthcare Organizations before the Committee on Health, Education, Labor and Pensions, U.S. Senate and the Subcommittee on Labor, Health and Human Services, and Education of the Senate Committee on Appropriations, Feb 22, 2000. Web site: *www.jcaho.org/govt/ oleary_022200.html.*

Chapter 1:

Preventing Operative and Postoperative Errors and Complications

Nowhere is the advance of contemporary medicine more apparent than in modern-day operating rooms and surgical suites. Once unimaginable feats, such as the permanent correction of vision and the simultaneous transplantation of multiple organs, occur daily if not routinely in thousands of ambulatory and hospital settings. Routine notwithstanding, error expert Marilyn Sue Bogner, PhD, calls the operating room a "hotbed for human error."[1] The environment is complex and dynamic, with constant change and time pressures. High-technology equipment is used extensively, as are potentially lethal drugs. Situational or environmental factors, including long working hours familiar to nurses in many care settings, impinge on human performance.

Operative procedures require the effort of physicians, nurses, and technicians working smoothly as a team. However, issues relevant to sentinel event prevention start well before the patient arrives in the operating room and later, in the postanesthesia recovery unit. With the extensive and increasing use of outpatient surgery, the nurse in the office or clinic and the nurse in the extended care facility might be involved in numerous prevention issues. This chapter addresses root causes and prevention strategies relevant throughout the care continuum for recipients of surgical care.

Cause for Concern

The past decades have witnessed a dramatic increase in the number and types of operative procedures. As operative volume increases, so does the risk of error and sentinel events. In a classic 1991 study, Lucian Leape and

colleagues with the Harvard Medical Practice Study analyzed all serious adverse events in hospitalized patients.[2] Although the research considered much more than sentinel events, Leape's data revealed that 48% of the adverse events were related to surgery. Wound infections were the most common surgical adverse event, accounting for 29% of surgical complications and nearly one-seventh of all adverse events identified in the study.

Leape's findings are very similar to those of the California Medical Association Study, conducted more than a decade earlier.[3] In this study, half the potential compensable events were found to result from treatment in the operating room. A study following Leape's indicated that about 20% of serious adverse events were related to surgery.[4] Data collected among health care consumers confirms the frequency of adverse events related to surgical or operative procedures. The public opinion poll conducted for the National Patient Safety Foundation found that 22% of patients surveyed had experienced mistakes during a medical (or surgical) procedure.[5]

Data from the Joint Commission's Sentinel Event database, including nearly 1,100 sentinel events reviewed by the organization from January 1995 through June 2001, indicates that operative and postoperative complications accounted for 12.5% of sentinel events. Wrong-site surgery accounted for 9.7%. When looked at cumulatively (22%), these sentinel events surpass all other types in occurrence frequency. A Sentinel Event Alert, published by the Joint Commission in 1998 on the topic of operative and postoperative complications, revealed that 84% of the sentinel event-related operative and postoperative complications documented by

---

Table 1-1. Most Frequent Operative or Postoperative Complications

- Insertion of nasogastric/feeding tubes into the trachea or a bronchus;

- Massive fluid overload during genitourinary/gynecological procedures due to the absorption of irrigation fluids;

- Acute respiratory failure and cardiac arrest during open orthopedic operations;

- Perforation of adjacent organs during endoscopic procedures, including nongastrointestinal procedures (for example, lacerations of the liver were among the most frequent complications of thoracic and abdominal endoscopic operations);

- Central venous catheter insertion into an artery;

- Liver lacerations, peritonitis, or respiratory arrest as the result of an imaging-directed percutaneous biopsy or tube placement; and

- Burns from electrocautery used with a flammable prep solution.

Source: Joint Commission: Operative and postoperative complications: Lessons for the future. *Sentinel Event Alert Issue* 12, Feb 4, 2000.

---

acute care hospitals resulted in deaths. Sixteen percent resulted in serious injury.[6] These data specifically excluded cases directly related to medication errors, the administration of anesthesia, and wrong-site surgery. The complications occurred during the induction of anesthesia (6%), intraoperatively (23%), during postanesthesia recovery (13%), and postoperatively (58%). Only 10% of the cases were considered emergencies. The procedures involved numerous specialties, including interventional imaging or endoscopy, tube or catheter insertion, open abdominal surgery, orthopedic surgery, head and neck surgery, and thoracic surgery. The most frequent complications appear as Table 1-1, above.

Since nurses are actively involved in all these stages and activities, they can contribute to preventing sentinel events in these areas.

Data related to wrong-site surgery are equally dramatic. For example, the American Academy of Orthopaedic Surgeons (AAOS) reports that, during the decade ending in 1995, 225 orthopedic wrong-site surgery claims were filed.[7] Most orthopedic errors occurred during arthroscopy and usually involved surgeons performing the correct procedure but on the wrong side. From 1979 to 2000, the Pennsylvania Medical Society Insurance Company paid out millions in claims

for 88 cases of wrong-site surgery involving such varied specialties as orthopedics, ophthalmology, neurosurgery, urology, and interventional radiology.[8]

Joint Commission data related to cases of wrong-site surgery were initially included in a *Sentinel Event Alert* published in 1998.[9] The cases involved orthopedic, urology, and neurosurgery procedures. However, wrong-site surgery is not limited to these specialties. Ophthalmology, interventional radiology, oral surgery, and general surgery can also be added to the list. No specialty can consider itself immune to the problem. Although most of the discussions involve the laterality aspects of operating on the wrong side, there also have been situations where the wrong procedure was done at the correct site or the correct procedure was done on the wrong patient.

Wrong-site surgery is always preventable. Traditionally, surgeons have had primary responsibility for ensuring that the correct site is being treated. However, root cause analyses of multiple wrong-site surgery cases demonstrates convincingly that multidisciplinary patient assessment and preparation coupled with communication among caregivers are the most critical functions and therefore, the locus of effective strategies for reducing the risk of wrong-site surgery. Caregivers (surgeons, anesthesiologists, and nurses) should always check the identity of the patient before beginning surgical procedures. Surgeons, anesthesiologists, and nurses take numerous precautions to prevent wrong-site surgery. But at times, even these measures have not prevented wrong-site surgery. It requires the cooperation and interdependence of all health care staff members including physicians, anesthesiologists, and nurses, as equal members of a team, to help reduce operative and postoperative errors.

The remainder of this chapter will focus on prevention strategies nurses may use working within a team environment to help reduce the likelihood of wrong-site surgery or other sentinel events resulting from operative and postoperative errors or complications.

Wrong-Site Surgery: Root Causes and Prevention Strategies

The causes of wrong-site surgery cross disciplinary boundaries and reflect systems failures. Joint Commission staff has identified several factors that increase the risk of a wrong-site situation:[9]

- More than one surgeon involved in the case, either because multiple procedures were contemplated or because the care of the patient was transferred to another surgeon.
- Multiple procedures were conducted on the same patient during a single trip to the operating room, especially when the procedures were on different sides of the patient's body.
- Unusual time pressures related to an unusual start time or pressure to speed up the preoperative procedures. These frequently involve staff-perceived time pressures.
- Unusual patient characteristics such as physical deformity or massive obesity that might alter the usual process for equipment set-up or positioning of the patient.

The Joint Commission's Sentinel Events database identifies root cause, systems-oriented error sources. Among the most frequently iden-

tified categories are the following: operating room (OR) team miscommunication; incomplete patient assessment; failure to follow organization's verification policy; OR hierarchy; lack of communication with patient; lack of verification process; necessary information not available in OR; distraction; and inadequate competence assessment/credentialing. A chart illustrating the percentage of wrong-site surgery errors attributed to each root cause appears as Figure 1-1, page 4. For most errors, multiple causes were identified. A thorough look at the root causes and responsibilities of nurses as team members is critical to the successful development and implementation of effective error prevention strategies.

Root Cause 1: Inadequate Communication

Sentinel Event Example: Communication Failure Among Caregiving Staff. *A review of a medical record by nursing staff indicates that a patient's history and physical examination (H&P) was completed by the patient's internist. The H&P notes that the patient has bilateral arthritis of both knees. The H&P concludes that the patient is scheduled for a total knee replacement, but there is no indication of which knee. The surgeon has no preoperative notes in the record because the patient had been admitted the day of the surgery. Because the patient does not speak English well, the nursing staff completes the informed consent based solely on information noted in the operating room schedule which calls for a right side total knee replacement. The surgery is performed on the wrong knee.*

"Near Miss" Example: Failure to Communicate Effectively with Patient and Family. *A surgeon's office staff mails informed consents to patients. Patients are instructed to sign the consent form and bring it to the hospital the day of surgery. An elderly patient receives the informed consent for a "cervical laminectomy with fusion." The woman does not recall the surgeon's mention of fusion. She calls her son who had accompanied her during the office visit when the surgery was discussed. The son, who is a physician, explains that not only was the "fusion" part wrong, but the procedure was to be a "lumbar laminectomy"—at the other end of the back.*

As illustrated by these examples, communication issues fall into two categories:

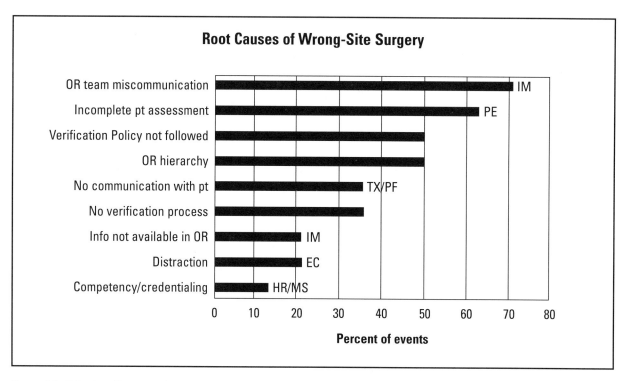

Figure 1-1. *This chart illustrates the percentage of causes at the root of wrong-site surgery errors reported to the Joint Commission between January 1995 and January 2001. The letters appearing at the end of each bar indicate relevant Joint Commission accreditation standard chapters.*

1. Communication among staff members: Inaccurate or incomplete communication among caregivers increases the risk of adverse events. At times, wrong-site surgery errors have occurred because certain members of the team are excluded from participation in the process for site verification or are hesitant to point out possible errors due to an intensely hierarchical culture. If the verification process relies solely on the surgeon's involvement, does the staff feel free to question his or her decision?

2. Communication with patient/family: Failure to involve the patient or family, where appropriate, in the process of identifying the correct site or procedure through the informed consent process can result in a wrong-site surgery.

Prevention Strategies

Communicate, communicate, communicate. Throughout the caregiving process, nurses must communicate to the next caregiver information concerning the site of surgery. Documentation in records is essential, but ver-bal communication helps to enhance information transfer. The operating room nurse should receive a report from the nurse caring for the patient, review relevant documentation, verify the information with the patient, and document the findings. In the operating room, the surgical team must be informed of the site of the procedure and participate in the verification process. Total reliance on the surgeon for verifying the site has been identified as problematic. In the office, clinic, or extended care facility, the patient's assessment and informed consent should be processed with pertinent details that indicate the exact site of the procedure. The method for communicating this information should be part of a formal, structured process.

Identify and communicate a flawed informed consent process. Nurses should continuously identify processes that can be improved. Many informed consent policies and procedures are elaborate, but fraught with pitfalls. Handling informed consent through the mail is one such process. As evident in the first example, completing the informed consent document without proper information in-hand presents enormous error risk. When the surgeon obtains informed consent during discussions with the patient and his or her family, for example, the nurse is not totally dependent on possibly erroneous information with which to complete consent forms. Nurses must ensure that consent is obtained before administering sedative medications.

Avoid using abbreviations when communicating about surgical sites and procedures. Spelling out "left" and "right" and the names of operative procedures helps to reduce confusion and the opportunity for error.

Root Cause 2: Incomplete Preoperative Patient Assessment

Sentinel Event Example: Inappropriate Assessment Procedure. *During particularly busy periods in a preoperative preparation and holding area, a nurse decides to streamline the process by filling in most of her preoperative nursing assessment form prior to the patient's arrival using information already in the patient's file. Instead of asking the patient the required assessment questions and comparing these data with the information gleaned from the record, for expediency's sake, the nurse skips over the areas already completed. Therefore, she does not avail herself of the opportunity to verify patient-provided information with other information in the chart.*

When an elderly patient arrives for a carpal tunnel procedure, the patient's escort is asked to remain in the waiting area. Unfortunately, the H&P does not indicate that the patient has some subtle memory problems, and a mental evaluation is not part of the nurse's evaluation. The surgery schedule has the wrong wrist specified for the surgery. The always-agreeing patient responds "Yes" to the nurse's question, "So we're performing the surgery on your left wrist, is that right?" The operation is performed on the wrong limb.

If the preoperative assessment had indicated the patient's memory problems, the nurse in this example would have realized that she could not use the patient's indication of laterality to confirm the site. In addition, rather than telling the patient the specific site, it is often useful to ask the question in a manner that requires the patient to state the site (that is, "Which hand are we operating on today?").

The lack of a thorough preoperative assessment of the patient is a frequent contributing factor to wrong-site surgery. Often, failure to review the medical record or imaging studies in the immediate preoperative period is involved. The site of the surgery and the surgical procedure must be clearly noted in the assessment. A "total knee replacement" statement in the chart does not indicate the side of the procedure. Laterality is often the key element in describing the surgical site.

Prevention Strategies

Ensure proper identification of the surgical site and procedure in each preoperative assessment. Asks questions if information is not clear. Nurses can help to ensure that each assessment includes identity of the site and the operative procedure, especially when multiple specialties are seeing the patient for multiple problems.

Ensure availability of critical information. Each preoperative assessment must include information from the informed consent, medical record, imaging studies, and other sources in verifying the site. Nurses should request such information if it is not available.

Root Cause 3: Faulty Operative Site, Procedure, and Patient Verification Process or Inadequate Information

"Near Miss" Example: Patient Verification. *Two outpatient surgery patients are sitting in the waiting area prior to having the same procedure on different limbs. The first name of one patient, "Morris," coincidentally is the same as the last name of the other patient. When the nurse enters the waiting area and calls, "Morris," the wrong patient follows the nurse to the wrong operating room. Fortunately, the nurse is trained to also ask for a birth date and social security number before applying an identification wristband. He identifies the error.*

"Near Miss" Example: Faulty Operative Site Verification Process. *A review of a postoperative medical record for a patient who had a craniotomy for a temporal lesion reveals that no preoperative identification of the side of the lesion took place. No site-verification information is included in the H&P, the*

nursing assessment, anesthesiology assessment, or the progress notes. The informed consent lists only "temporal craniotomy." The only mention of the lesion site (left versus right) appears on one radiology report. The organization has no operative site verification process. Only the surgeon verifies the site in the operating room. The patient did fine, but a wrong-site surgery error could easily have occurred.

Sentinel Event Example: Failed Operative Site Verification Process. *A nurse verifies with a male patient that his arthroscopic surgery is for the right knee. This correlates with the posting and the consent form. The surgeon talks with the patient in the holding area and places a dot above the patient's left knee, thereby marking the wrong knee. Neither the nurse nor the surgeon communicate in the operating room about the procedure site. The surgeon operates on the wrong knee of the now anesthetized patient.*

These examples illustrate the importance of a thorough verification process to guarantee that the correct patient is matched with the correct procedure and that the correct operative site is identified. Such procedures often are flawed due to the absence of one or more factors including: a formal procedure; involvement of the patient in the verification procedure; a final check in the operating room; oral communication in the verification process; relevant information in the operating room; and a checklist to guarantee that all information has been reviewed.[9] The wrong-site surgery occurring in the third example could have been prevented by a step in the verification procedures that required pre-incision verification of the correct site by each team member. The verification technique should require oral verification of the correct site in the operating room by each member of the team. A list of people and items that should participate in or can be used in the verification process appear in Table 1-2, page 7.

In some instances surveyed by the Joint Commission and reported in the literature, the wrong procedure was performed at the correct site. This sentinel event reflects a failure to verify the procedure, perhaps due to the lack of adequate information in the operating room. The need for an exacting but workable policy regarding the identification of the procedure and site of surgery requires a multidisciplinary,

collaborative effort. From the initial scheduling of the procedure, to its actual performance, multiple people are involved in this complex endeavor. The nursing staff is well positioned to lead the site and procedure-verification effort because of its involvement in so many of the key process steps.

Prevention Strategies

Understand the verification policy and process. Several nurses are usually involved in preparing the patient for surgery. Responsibilities may vary considerably, but everyone involved must understand the process for identifying the correct surgical site. Staffing levels and staff orientation, training, and competence assessment play a major role in root causes of wrong-site surgery. Organization leaders must ensure enough personnel with proper orientation and training to follow the established policies and procedures. Staff must be properly trained in the appropriate verification techniques and recognize unacceptable practices. Staff competence in verification policies and procedures must be evaluated on a regular basis.

Take an active role in verifying the proper patient and surgical site. The nurse preparing the patient for surgery should review all the information provided, including the H&P, informed consent, X-rays, the operating room schedule, and any other available information. In addition, the nurse should verbally verify the site with the patient and/or family. Any conflicting information should be resolved immediately. Documentation should be complete and exact. The nurse's assessment should be compared with other assessments. Multiple assessments by several disciplines provide additional opportunities to identify the correct site. The nurses in the operating room have similar responsibilities. As mentioned earlier, the verification process should require oral verification of the correct site in the operating room by each team member.

Know the rules concerning H&Ps and ensure their thorough review. Nurses should be knowledgeable about who is permitted to perform a H&P and the period for which it is acceptable, and review the document for accuracy. A note that merely

---

Table 1-2. People and Items That Can Be Helpful to the Verification Process

People who can verify the surgical site:
- Patient and/or family
- RN on the nursing unit
- RN in the preoperative holding area
- Circulating RN
- Surgeon
- Anesthesiologist and/or certified registered nurse anesthetist

Documentation that can be used to verify the surgical site:
- Procedure schedule
- Operative consent
- History and physical
- Nursing assessment
- Preanesthesia assessment
- X-ray films and reports
- Surgeon's office notes
- A "mark" on the site
- Site checklist

Some of these people or items may not apply in every case. Each organization should determine consistent elements in the verification process.

---

indicates "H&P dictated" is not a useful document. In one egregious case, a surgeon felt that he could submit the same H&P that he had used for the patient three weeks earlier when the patient had a different procedure. Obviously, if the surgeon does not update the findings, the listed procedure will be wrong, and therefore useless in verifying the procedure site.

Know the policy and procedure for marking the site. If an organization's verification process requires marking the site, leaders must determine who is to mark the site, when the site is to be marked, and how the site is to be marked. The nurse must be aware of how this activity is to be accomplished. The policy for marking the site must be precise and consistent, or the marking becomes useless, and possibly dangerous. If one physician uses an "X" to indicate the site, but another surgeon uses "X" to denote "not the site," then the process is fraught with peril. The AAOS recommends that the surgeon clearly

mark the operative site with a surgical pen, signing his or her name directly on the operative site.[10] The AAOS points out that marking the non-surgical limb with the word "no" is not useful since the non-surgical limb will not be visible when the patient is draped. The surgeon should not proceed unless the marking is visible. Nurses and other OR team members should never assume the signature is under the drapes. Communication by nurses when surgeons do not follow organization protocols can help to reduce the likelihood of error.

Help ensure the use and availability of critical information in the operating room. Nurses can facilitate this process by helping to ensure that notes are available to the surgeon. One strategy suggested by experts to help reduce the likelihood of an error involving the wrong procedure performed at the correct site is to place the patient's chart on a stand in the operating room, and open it to the surgeon's notes describing the planned procedure. The surgeon could then quickly review the record prior to beginning.

Ensure use of thorough checklists. Nurses can use a verification checklist to ensure the review of all relevant documents as part of the operative site verification process. This list could include the clinical record, imaging reports, the informed consent, the operating room schedule and record, the anesthesia pre-assessment record, and direct observation of the marked operative site. A description of a thorough checklist system used by some organizations appears in Sidebar 1-1, page 9.

Two steps frequently are missing from checklist use. The first step is reviewing the information in reports and assessments for *content.* This obviously goes beyond simply noting the *presence* of the various reports and assessments. The second step involves ensuring agreement from all team members about the information collected, and not simply checking the information independently.

Operative and Postoperative Complications: Root Causes and Prevention Strategies

As with wrong-site surgery, the causes of sentinel events due to all other operative and postoperative errors and complications cross disciplinary boundaries and reflect systems failures. Organizations experiencing operative and postoperative sentinel events reviewed by the Joint Commission to-date identified the following as root causes:[6]

- Incomplete communication among caregivers;
- Failure to follow established procedures;
- Necessary personnel not being available when needed;
- Incomplete preoperative assessment;
- Deficiencies in credentialing and privileging;
- Inadequate supervision of house staff;
- Inconsistent postoperative monitoring procedures; and
- Failure to question inappropriate orders.

A review of key root causes and the responsibilities of nurses as team members are critical to the successful development and implementation of effective error prevention strategies.

Root Cause 1: Insufficient Caregiver Communication

Sentinel Event Example: Insufficient Sharing of Information. *A patient has a central venous line inserted while waiting in his hospital room prior to going to the operating room. The surgical resident orders a chest x-ray to determine the position of the catheter. Before the results of the x-ray are available, the surgical resident has to leave the area to attend to a serious situation in the emergency room. After the patient is sent to the operating room, the unit clerk on the patient's floor receives the radiology report, and posts the report in the patient's box. The report indicates the presence of a dangerous pneumothorax.*

The information concerning the pneumothorax is not sent to the operating room because radiology does not communicate the urgency of the report. The unit clerk does not know what information should be directed to the operating room. The staff in the operating room does not note that a piece of vital information is missing. Due to these factors, the patient suffers a cardiopulmonary arrest during the procedure.

This example demonstrates the critical importance of well-established communication channels, and the need to prioritize information sent and received. Two-thirds of the organizations reporting sentinel events due to operative/postoperative errors and complications to the Joint Commission identified incomplete communication among caregivers as a root cause. Usually a patient undergoing an operative procedure comes into contact with multiple members of an organization's staff and health care providers in the community. Nursing leaders can foster communication among providers and ensure the transfer of information among health care workers. They help create a climate that is conducive to a team approach. This climate must be supported by all organization leaders.

Organization leaders also must clearly define expected channels of communication. Direct communication among health care providers is

SIDEBAR 1-1. DESCRIPTION OF A VERIFICATION CHECKLIST

Some facilities have developed a checklist that includes both the documents and the personnel involved in the case. The form has three columns: the components being checked, a column titled RIGHT, and column titled LEFT. The person examining a document initials the correct box indicating the side recorded in the document. A person marking the site, or questioning the patient, initials the appropriate box. Each health care provider marks the site they have discussed with the patient. The checklist can be started by anyone, at any point in the process. Finally, in the operating room, the circulating nurse checks for any items not addressed, documents that all the initialed boxes are in the same column, and announces to the surgeon the site indicated by the checklist. If any initialed box is not consistent with the other boxes, then the process is halted until the situation is clarified. Discrepancies in the checklist are readily apparent.

obviously the optimal method for preventing mishaps. But because it is not always possible, the need for other accurate and precise methods of communication must be considered and developed. Many organizations have found that the use of multidisciplinary progress notes improves communication among health care providers and makes care plans more useful. By having all the information in the same area of the record, it is easier to identify what is incomplete or missing. Multidisciplinary progress notes also increase the relevance and use of the care plans.

Often different departments or divisions develop forms to document their activities. However, department outsiders may not be able to interpret the comments, abbreviations, or terminology used in the form. Efforts to standardize terminology, definitions, vocabulary, nomenclature, abbreviations, and symbols should be undertaken. Failure to do so invites error. A table that provides abbreviations, symbols and their meaning could be kept with patients' clinical records for ease of reference.

Through thorough documentation, the nurse provides a record that can be used to recognize problems or develop improvements. Documentation aids communication. For example, often a nurse must communicate to a physician information from a radiology report that confirms the correct placement of a catheter.

Failure to communicate the results of a confirmation procedure has led to misplacement of tubes and catheters. The confirmation report also may be sent to a long term care facility if the patient is transferred shortly after the catheter placement. Communication through this document enhances care continuity throughout the continuum of care. The requirement for an operative progress note to be entered immediately in the medical record after surgery reduces the likelihood of postoperative complications. Properly documented care plans help to ensure communication to all caregivers and optimal patient care.

Prevention Strategies

Use documentation as a communication tool. Educating personnel about the information in forms used by other disciplines makes documents useful communication tools. Nurses at one organization asked the anesthesia department to present an in-service lecture that would teach the nurses how to read the anesthesia record and preoperative assessment sheet. By being able to interpret the anesthesia record, they were able to follow specific events, review vital signs, identify medications and fluids used, and understand plans for the recovery period.

Use clinical practice guidelines to enhance communication. When available and appropriate, clinical practice guidelines provide a means to improve care quality and communication and enhance utilization of health care services. Guideline use requires all care team members to consider and understand the overall clinical process and the serial and parallel events that must be accomplished to complete a task or procedure. Practice guidelines offer an excellent opportunity to guarantee that the needed communication issues are addressed. When designing clinical processes or checking the design of existing processes, communication should be considered at each step, using the communication tools that complement the activities.

Question inappropriate orders. Nurses must feel comfortable enough about established communication channels to promptly and freely question orders that they feel may be inappropriate or unclear. A hierarchical approach to medical care must be replaced by a teamwork approach. Leaders should encourage frank and respectful communication among team players and not tolerate intimidation of any member of the health care team. Direct communication between physicians and other health care providers is key to the prevention of sentinel events due to operative complications.

Root Cause 2: Failure to Follow Established Policies and Procedures

Sentinel Event Example: Foregoing Procedure.

A busy surgeon requests that a new prep solution be added to the stock of solutions used during operative procedures. The prep solution's information insert indicates that the solution is flammable unless allowed to dry. The organization's operating room procedures require an in-service presentation of any new product, procedure, or piece of equipment prior to use. When the surgeon asks for the solution in the operating room, she is informed that although the product is available, she will not be able to use it because the nurses have not yet received training related to its use. She questions the need for a class on something as simple as a prep solution, and forcefully asks for the solution. Although the nurses question the surgeon's request, they are intimidated and agree to her demands.

The circulating nurse preps the patient's neck with the new solution, and the surgeon quickly steps forward and drapes the patient. The nurse does not have the opportunity to remove the towels placed on either side

of the neck to catch prep solution drippings. The presence of towels containing the pooled solution makes the situation extremely dangerous. The surgeon makes a skin incision using an electrocautery knife. The site and the drapes burst into flames. The patient suffers serious burns on his neck, chest, and face.

The surgeon and the operating staff in this example lacked the knowledge necessary to use the new product safely. They had not received the required training session, as per organization policy. Half of the organizations experiencing a sentinel event related to an operative or postoperative error reported to the Joint Commission since 1995 identified a failure to follow policies as one root cause. Physicians, nurses, and other OR team members must be trained and expected to follow established procedures at all times. Joint Commission Care of the Patient standards address the selection of appropriate procedures, preparation of the patient for the procedures, execution of the procedures, patient monitoring, and postoperative care.

Prevention Strategies

Be knowledgeable about organizational policies and procedures. Organization leaders establish policies and procedures in order to reduce the risk of adverse events. The design of procedures must take into account human factors such as the tendency to take short cuts. Policies and procedures must be available to nurses so that they know what is expected of them. Education about policies and procedures provides nurses with an understanding of how the policy or procedure effectively prevents sentinel events. Leaders must ensure that nurses are complying with established policies and procedures. Nurses must ensure their own compliance and help ensure the compliance of other members of the interdisciplinary team.

Monitor consistency of compliance with procedures. Because of the critical importance of following policies and procedures, nurse managers should collect and analyze compliance data. When performance is inconsistent, managers must evaluate the process to determine whether the procedure's design lends itself to compliance errors, and why. Some nursing directors establish a regular routine for observing the performance of specific procedures, particularly those associated with high risks.

Standardize procedures across care settings. Nursing leaders must help to ensure uniform performance of patient care processes. The frequently stated principle "one level of care" recognizes the importance of standardized policies and procedures. A collaborative, multidisciplinary approach to standardization across various settings enables collaborative learning, decreases confusion during training, and establishes consistent performance evaluation methods. For example, due to high complication rates, one organization recognized the need to standardize the procedure for inserting central-line catheters. Following implementation of a redesigned policy, consistent training, and standardized equipment, the organization significantly improved the complication rate experienced throughout the facility. Use of standardized procedures for other high risk activities such as conscious sedation, emergency care, pain management, and hyperalimentation helps to reduce the likelihood of adverse events.

Root Cause 3: Inadequate Competence Assessment, Credentialing, or Staffing

Sentinel Event Example: Inadequate Training.

An orthopedic surgeon, covering one evening for his partner, arrives in an emergency room to care for a patient with a dislocated shoulder. The surgeon rarely performs elective procedures at this facility. He states that he intends to use conscious sedation while setting the patient's shoulder. The emergency room nurse is aware that the hospital recently instituted a program for physician training, testing, and privileging in conscious sedation. One of the topics taught in the program is the ability to assess risk prior to instituting conscious sedation. The patient's obese stature and problems with sleep apnea are clear indicators that the patient is at increased risk for an adverse outcome. However, there is no mechanism in the emergency room to verify the physician's privileges in conscious sedation. The surgeon assures the nurse that he is competent in the use of conscious sedation. He commences the procedure. The patient experiences a respiratory arrest.

A review of the surgeon's credentials and privileges reveals that he did not attend the hospital's training program and was not privileged at the facility for conscious sedation.

Organizations experiencing sentinel events related to operative and postoperative procedures frequently cite clinical competence and credentialing and staff orientation, training, and availability as root causes. Although medical staff leaders determine clinical privileges, the nursing staff should know how to determine if a physician has been granted the privileges he or she intends to perform. The nurse in this example could have specifically asked the physician whether he had attended the new conscious sedation program.

Staff training, competence, and adequacy are leadership issues. An adequate number of staff members with the experience and training necessary must be available to meet patient care needs. The special training required for various operations or procedures makes staffing a challenge in most hospitals and ambulatory settings.

Many organizations maintain generic competencies lists and job descriptions for categories of employees. These do not meet the requirements outlined in Joint Commission Human Resource standards. Job descriptions and competence requirements must accurately reflect the job being performed. Accurate and specific requirements serve as guidelines for orientation, training, and competence assessment. Nursing leaders must continuously assess competence, collect and analyze data on competence patterns, and determine staff learning needs. The data collection must be based on a meaningful competence evaluation process that assesses each staff member's ability to meet performance expectations outlined in his or her job description. Generic evaluation forms can assess only the basics. Specific tasks, especially those involving procedures and equipment, must be evaluated. Assessment of age-specific competence must include actual observation of specific tasks related to the patients involved.

Prevention Strategies

Ensure appropriate credentials and privileges of practitioners performing procedures. When a physician or other practitioner arrives on a unit requesting to perform an invasive procedure, the nursing staff should have a mechanism for identifying privileges held by that practitioner. Although this places the nursing staff in an often uncomfortable position, timely checking can help prevent sentinel events. During the day, a nurse manager can usually check with the medical staff office. However, in the evening, that might not be possible. As the patient's advocate, nursing supervisors must help to ensure that those performing procedures are qualified to do so.

Inform supervisor of unsafe staffing situations. Again, as patient advocates, nurses must communicate their concern about unsafe staffing situations. Notification of a supervisor and documentation of the situation through whatever mechanism is available in the organization are appropriate. Nurses should feel comfortable about reporting their concerns every time they encounter the situation.

Ensure that job descriptions and competence requirements accurately reflect the job being performed. Nurse directors or managers must ensure that they are evaluating the performance of actual skills and tasks performed by nurses on the job. The nurses themselves can help make sure this happens by keeping managers informed of their daily activities and changes in these activities. As new competencies emerge, these must be added to the assessment process for each nurse performing the skill or task.

Root Cause 4: Inadequate Preoperative Assessment and Postoperative Monitoring Procedures

Sentinel Event Example: Incomplete Preoperative Assessment. *During an endoscopy nurse's preoperative assessment of a patient scheduled for a colonoscopy, the patient reveals that he is also scheduled for a cardiac stress test three days later. The patient does not recall why he is having the stress test. The nurse fails to bring this information to the gastroenterologist's attention prior to the procedure.*

Following the colonoscopy, the patient develops chest pain in the recovery room and is diagnosed with a myocardial infarction. The committee reviewing this complication determines that this patient's preoperative assessment was incomplete. The procedure should have been rescheduled pending stress test results.

"Near Miss" Example: Faulty Postoperative Monitoring. *During a shoulder reduction in the emergency department, an obese twenty-five year old requires a considerable amount of narcotics and benzodiazopines for pain control. In the recovery period, the lack of stimulation causes a decrease in his ventilation, with a decrease in oxygen saturation. The patient is then given reversal agents for both the narcotics and benzodazopines. Shortly thereafter, the patient is awake, alert, and has normal oxygen saturation levels.*

However, since the facility does not have a policy indicating how long the patient should be monitored after the use of a reversal agent, the patient is discharged from the recovery period in the emergency department 10 minutes later. Since the narcotics in the patient's system last longer than the reversal agent, the patient becomes renarcotized at home and is brought back to the emergency department by ambulance. He experiences increased sedation and an altered breathing pattern. Staff stabilize him and he is able to return home six hours later.

The lack of a complete preoperative assessment is one of the root causes associated with various operative adverse events. The events might be the result of missing information concerning laboratory data, the existence and status of pre-existing diseases, and changes in the patient's health. The lack of information might be reflected in an inappropriate choice of an anesthetic or a surgical procedure, the decision to use or not use a medication, and the failure to plan appropriately for the postoperative period. Examples of possible adverse events include

- failure to recognize the patient on anticoagulants prior to invasive procedures, resulting in bleeding situations;

- failure to recognize the patient with sleep apnea, resulting in a serious respiratory response with sedation; and

- failure to identify the patient with a medication allergy, resulting in an anaphylactic reaction.

The nurse should not only observe that the pre-assessment is present, but also review the assessment in depth to identify questionable or confusing information.

In the area of postoperative monitoring, the Joint Commission requires that patients be monitored continuously during the postoperative period. Monitoring should include

■ physiological and mental status;

■ status of or findings related to pathological conditions, such as drainage from incisions;

■ intravenous fluids and drugs administered, including blood and blood components;

■ impairments and functional status;

■ pain intensity and quality, and responses to treatments; and

■ unusual events or postoperative complications and their management.

Often various categories of patients come through an operating room's postanesthesia care unit (PACU). Outpatients, inpatients, and same-day-admit patients should receive postoperative monitoring. Organization policies should address any differences in required monitoring. In some circumstances, a patient might be transferred directly from the operating room to an intensive care unit (ICU). Is the immediate postoperative care comparable to the PACU care? Are ICU and PACU nurses similarly trained for immediate postoperative care? The staff member responsible for the patient's immediate postprocedural care should be identified. In the PACU, anesthesiologists are directly responsible for the patient until discharged from the recovery room. ICU nurses should know who to contact with the results of the laboratory tests and changes in vital signs, and to evaluate the patient. The staff member responsible for the patient's care during the immediate postoperative period in the ICU should be clear.

Often procedures with and without conscious sedation are done in numerous places in a facility. A consistent policy should be in place throughout the facility for postoperative monitoring in sites outside the operating room's PACU. In one facility, patients who had procedures completed in the endoscopy suite fell into two categories: outpatients were transferred to the PACU for monitoring and eventual discharge, and inpatients were discharged directly to their hospital rooms. A comparison of the two groups revealed that inpatients received minimal postoperative monitoring.

Organization leaders must develop and implement policies and procedures addressing each of the questions raised above.

Prevention Strategies

Ensure that preoperative assessments are available and accurate. Nurses can help guarantee that needed assessments are available and accurate. The nurse should be familiar with the scope of the components required in the H&P, the nursing assessment, and consultant assessments. Familiarity with assessment time frames as specified in organization policies, health care providers who can provide the assessments, and special requirements for anesthesia enable the nurse to identify assessment portions that are incomplete and identify opportunities to improve the process.

Compare available information to ensure consistency of data. In addition to identifying incomplete assessment sections, the nurse can also compare the information available in the assessments, laboratory reports, and various forms to ensure the consistency of data. By identifying the pieces that do not match, corrective steps can be achieved before a serious situation develops. Often nurses are in the best position to help select the forms and technology that will enhance gathering and presentation of required information.

Know and follow the organization's postoperative monitoring policies. The key strategy in achieving satisfactory postoperative monitoring is for the nursing staff to become familiar with postoperative monitoring policies through thorough training, orientation, and competence assessment. Collaborative efforts of the various departments involved in determining the postoperative monitoring policies and procedures will help ensure the identification and implementation of the best possible policies.

Use high quality monitoring documentation forms. A monitoring documentation form reminds the nurse what activities and documentation must be completed. Forms should clearly identify the elements to be monitored, the time periods involved, and discharge criteria. Documentation that consists of long, written comments is often difficult to review, and often has pieces missing. A well-organized form can be very useful to both the recorder and the reviewer. Often, items can be recorded using numbers or letters that correspond to specific definitions (such as the different levels of consciousness). A graphic representation is often used to indicate the basic vital signs. An example of a documentation form used by one organization is provided as Figure 1-2, page 15.

Understand how to use collected data. In addition to knowing what to monitor, the nurses must understand how to use the collected data. Video tests can be used to evaluate training programs. By using simulators or computer programs to alter the variables being monitored, the staff can be trained to respond to numerous situations.

Closing Comments

Nurses can play a significant role in reducing the likelihood of sentinel events associated with operative complications or errors and wrong-site surgery. Prevention strategies address and span the breadth of challenges to safe health care. These include incomplete assessment, failure to follow established policies, inadequate staff training or competence assessment, and insufficient communication or information availability. To empower nurses to make a difference, leaders must ensure a collaborative environment conducive to thorough multidisciplinary communication.

References

1. Bogner MS (ed): *Human Error in Medicine.* Hillsdale, NJ: Lawrence Erlbaum Associates, 1994, p 378.

2. Leape LL, et al: The nature of adverse events in hospitalized patients: Results of the Harvard Medical Practice Study. *New England Journal of Medicine* 324:377–384, 1991.

3. California Medical Association: Report of the Medical Insurance Feasibility Study. San Francisco: California Medical Association, 1977.

4. Andrews LB, et al: An alternative strategy for studying adverse events in medical care. *Lancet* 349:309–313, 1997.

5. National Patient Safety Foundation at the American Medical Association: *Public Opinion of Patient Safety Issues: Research Findings.* Sep 1997. Web site: *www.npsf.org.*

6. Joint Commission: Operative and postoperative complications: Lessons for the future. *Sentinel Event Alert* Issue 12, Feb 4, 2000.

7. Joint Commission: *Using Hospital Standards to Prevent Sentinel Events,* Oakbrook Terrace, IL: Joint Commission, 2001, p 70.

8. Prager L: Mishaps rare, but 100% preventable, surgeons group says. *Los Angeles Times Syndicate* Nov 18, 1998.

9. Joint Commission: Lessons learned: Wrong-site surgery. *Sentinel Event Alert* Issue 6, Aug 28, 1998.

10. Healthcare Risk Management: Confirm correct site, then apply your John Hancock, March 1999, p 31.

Clarian Health
Methodist IU Riley

Intra-Procedure and Post Procedure Assessment

Scheduled Procedure: _____   Actual Procedure:_____

Start Time: _____   Stop Time: _____   IV Fluid: _____   Total Given: _____

Medications:	Dosage/ Route	Time/ Initials	Dosage/ Route	Time/ Initials	Dosage/ Route	Time/ Initials	Dosage/ Route	Time/ Initials	Totals

Vital Signs:

Time	BP	HR	RR	O$_2$Sat	O$_2$	Level of Sedation*	Comments	Initials
							Baseline Data	

Legend: *Level of Sedation
1-Fully awake, alert, appropriate for age or pre-sedation level
2-Sedated but awake

3-Sleeping, arouses to verbal stimuli
4-Sleeping, arouses to physical stimuli
5-Does not respond to stimuli

RA=Room air
NC=Nasal canula
TC=Tracheal collar

Criteria for Discharge/Return to Routine Monitoring			**Post-Procedure Instructions**
Patient Met Criteria or Has Returned to Baseline:	YES	NO	**Inpatient:** Return to Unit: _____
Level of Consciousness	❑	❑	Report Called:_____ AM/PM Initials: _____
Usual mobility or as appropriate per procedure	❑	❑	Remains on Unit:_____
BP +/– 29mm of pre-sedation level	❑	❑	RN receiving report: _____
Pulse 60–100 adults/80–140 peds, rhythm regular	❑	❑	**Outpatient:** Written Discharge Instructions:_____
RR 12–20 >3 yrs/20–40 <3yrs, normal pattern	❑	❑	_____
O^2 Sat >90% or equal to pre-sedation	❑	❑	_____
Swallows PO fluids, secretions or + gag reflex	❑	❑	
Pt can progress to previous monitoring level	❑	❑	❑ Given to pt ❑ Given to Responsible Person/Driver

Signatures:	**Initials**	Comments:_____
		_____
		_____

Pt. Released by:_____   Released to:_____   Time:_____AM/PM

Figure 1-2. *This assessment documentation form, provided by Clarion Health Partners in Indianapolis, includes key information necessary to effectively monitor a patient during and after a procedure.*

Chapter 2:

Preventing Medication Errors

In all health care settings—the hospital, home, long term care or assisted living facility, behavioral health, or ambulatory facility—we hear echoes of phrases like, "The nurse gave the medication without question." These words are followed frequently by an example of a serious medication error leading to a negative outcome for the individual receiving care, at times resulting in an unexpected death or serious injury. Although this medication error actually may have originated several steps back in the medication use process when the physician wrote the order or the pharmacist filled the order, the nurse frequently receives blame for making the error since he or she administered the medication. This chapter examines root causes and prevention strategies for medication errors that originate with the nurse, and those coming to the nurse from an earlier place in the medication use process, which he or she could play a role in preventing at the point of administration.

The Medication Use System

To understand how nurses can help prevent medication errors, we look first at the medication use system itself, which provides the framework for drug therapy for all individuals receiving care. The medication use system in all types of health care facilities and in the home setting is very complex, often involving dozens of separate yet interrelated, if not sequential, steps. With the recent introduction of electronic ordering, bar coding, and advanced decentralized dispensing technology, U.S. health care is now on the threshold of a new medication use era.

An expert panel convened by the Joint Commission defined the medication use system

as, "the safe, effective, appropriate, and efficient use of medications."[1] It commences with drug selecting and procuring by an interdisciplinary team, including clinicians and administrators, and advances through drug prescribing by the practitioner; drug preparation and dispensing by the pharmacist; drug administering by the nursing and other health professional staff; and drug therapy monitoring by the nursing, medical, and pharmacy staffs (see Figure 2-1, page 18). One or more of these stages occur in most organizations providing health care services. The five processes share the common goal of safe, effective, appropriate, and efficient provision of drug therapy to individuals receiving care. The objective is to provide the "six rights"—the *right* dose of the *right* drug to the *right* individual via or by the *right* route at the *right* time with the *right* results.

Medication errors are frequently categorized and studied according to when they occur in the medication use process. For example, one study found that 39% of serious medication errors occurred in the prescribing process, 50% in the order transcription and drug administration processes, and 11% during the dispensing process.[2] Errors frequently involve multiple stages of the drug use process. This primarily is due to the fact that the medication use function involves many different types of health care professionals, each interacting at different points in the medication use function. When professionals work together as interdependent and equally essential team members, medication errors can effectively be reduced.

Deborah M. Nadzam, PhD, RN, administrative director of the Quality Institute at the Cleveland Clinic Health System and a key contact for the National Coordinating Council for Medication

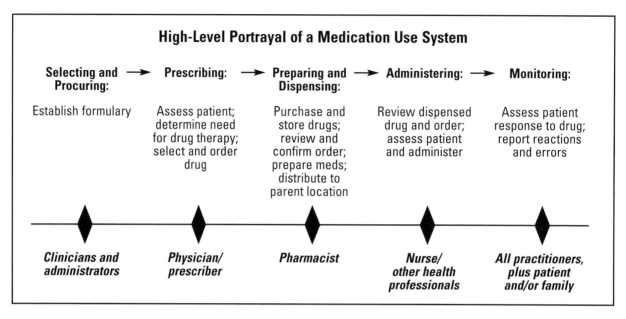

Figure 2-1. *This chart, developed by an expert panel convened by the Joint Commission to define the medication use function, depicts the overall processes and individuals involved in the medication use system in an acute care environment.*

Error Reporting and Prevention, describes traditional medication use team members as follows:[1]

■ *Administrators and clinicians* are at the "front-end" of the process, making decisions regarding the selection, procurement, and storage of drugs according to care and organization needs. They establish formularies, direct the development and implementation of staff education programs, and identify and procure necessary equipment, among other functions.

■ *Physicians and other health care prescribers* assess the individual receiving care to determine the appropriate drug therapy, select and order the appropriate drug(s) and therapeutic regimen, and monitor the individual's clinical condition to determine the effect of the drug. Prescribers reevaluate the drug selection, regimen, frequency, and duration, as necessary.

■ *Pharmacists* procure, store, prepare, and dispense medications and provide information to other professionals regarding established and new drug therapies. They ensure correct labeling and timely and accurate dispensing. In their role as reviewers of all drug orders and prescriptions, they question unusual dosages, routes of administration, and frequencies.

■ *Nurses,* a term used for many different types of professionals, including licensed practical nurses, registered nurses, clinical nurse specialists, and nurse practitioners, administer medications and are in frequent contact with the individuals receiving care. Thus, they are able to note negative side effects. Although typically unable to administer medications, nursing aides also observe individuals and note side effects. Nurses serve as the final check to ensure that the pharmacy has delivered what the prescriber ordered and that the order appears appropriate given the individual's condition, allergies, and other factors. They assess the individual receiving care to determine whether a change in condition warrants withholding the medication. They increasingly are becoming active participants in the entire medication use process.

■ *Individuals receiving care,* the recipients of medications, and *families or significant others* participate in medication administration and monitoring activities. In the Internet age, familiarity with medications is increasing as stays in health care settings shorten and more care is provided at home. Health care professionals must make the individuals receiving care and their caregivers partners in the medication use process.

All team members play a significant role in reducing the likelihood of medication errors.

Medication Error Defined

A *medication error* is defined by the National Coordinating Council for Medication Error Reporting and Prevention (NCC MERP), an independent body comprised of 19 national organizations, including the Joint Commission, as

> any preventable event that may cause or lead to inappropriate medication use or patient harm while the medication is in the control of the health care professional, patient, or consumer. Such events may be related to professional practice, health care products, procedures, and systems, including prescribing; order communication; product labeling, packaging, and nomenclature; compounding; dispensing; distribution; administration; education; monitoring; and use.[3]

Health care literature is full of other closely related terms that warrant definition as well, including adverse drug event, adverse drug reaction, and medication misadventure. An *adverse drug event* (ADE) is an injury resulting from a medication or lack of an intended medication.[4,5] An *adverse drug reaction* (ADR) is any unexpected, unintended, undesired, or excessive response to a drug, with or without an "injury."[5] An ADR negatively affects prognosis and may result in temporary or permanent harm, disability, or death. It may or may not be the result of a medication error, such as with a medication side effect. Response to an ADR may require a range of actions, including admitting an individual to a health care facility, providing supportive treatments, discontinuing the medicine, changing the medication therapy, or modifying the dose.

This book focuses on strategies to prevent medication errors that, through omission or commission, lead to or could lead to injury.

Cause for Concern

Medication errors occur with alarming frequency. Although *in*frequently resulting in death or serious injury, those medication errors that *do* shake the foundation of public confidence in health care and increase health care costs. In fact, the results of a national survey indicate that worries about drug errors dominate care recipient concerns about visits to health care organizations.[6] Of the top five concerns expressed by care recipients, being given the wrong medicine ranks number one, being given two or more medicines that interact in a negative way ranks number two, and not having enough information about the medicines they receive ranks number five. A 1997 public opinion survey conducted for the National Patient Safety Foundation found that medication errors ranked number two in types of mistakes experienced by respondents, with 28% indicating that they experienced a medication error in a health care setting.[7]

Estimates of the occurrence of medication errors and adverse drug events vary widely. The often-cited 1995 study by David W. Bates and his colleagues at Brigham and Women's Hospital and Massachusetts General Hospital indicates an adverse drug event rate of 6.5 events per 100 nonobstetrical admissions to hospitals.[8] Donald Berwick, president and CEO of the Institute for Healthcare Improvement, estimates that medication errors affect between 20% and 40% of all medication doses.[9] A review of death certificates, described in the 1999 IOM report, showed that 7,391 people died in one recent year from medication errors acknowledged by health care personnel or care recipients.[10] This level of suffering and loss is tragic and avoidable.

Types of Medication Errors

In 1998, NCC MERP published the "NCC MERP Taxonomy of Medication Errors" to be used in combination with systems analysis in recording and tracking of medication errors. Medication error types identified by the organization appear in Figure 2-2, page 20.

Root Causes and Prevention Strategies

The causes of medication errors cross disciplinary boundaries reflecting systems failures outlined in Table 2-1, page 18. The Joint

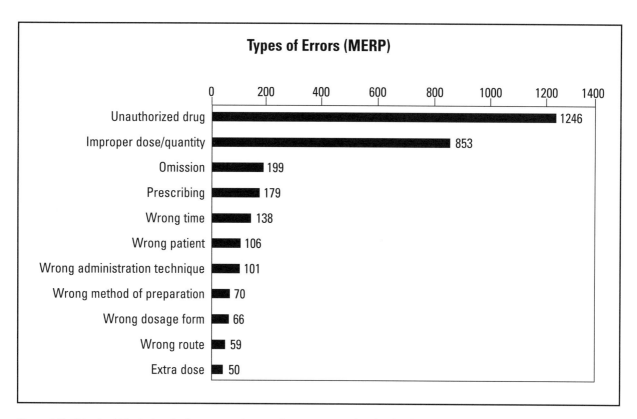

Figure 2-2. *This chart illustrates the frequency of types of errors reported to the database of the USP Medication Errors Reporting Program (MERP) over the five-year period 1995–1999.* **Source:** *U.S. Pharmacopeia. Used with permission.*

Commission's Sentinel Events database provides one categorization for root cause, systems-oriented error sources. Among the most frequently identified categories are the following: orientation/training; communication; storage/access; information availability; competency/credentialing; supervision; labeling; and distraction. A chart illustrating the percentage of medication errors reported to the Joint Commission since January of 1995 attributed to each root cause appears as Figure 2-3, page 22. Note that for most medication errors, multiple root causes were identified.

Other categorizations are helpful as well. The major cause and contributing factors categories outlined in the *NCC MERP Taxonomy of Medication Errors* appear by frequency of occurrence for a sampling of errors reported to the MedMARx, the U.S. Pharmacopeia's Internet-accessible database, in Figure 2-4, page 23.

A thorough look at each root cause, as identified by the Joint Commission, and the roles and responsibilities of nurses as team members are critical both to developing a systems approach

to error prevention and targeting improvement opportunities. The remaining sections in this book focus on the role the nurse plays in preventing medication errors and implementing proactive safety strategies for frequently occurring root causes.

Root Cause 1: Inadequate Orientation, Training, or Education

Sentinel Event Example: Failure to Follow Policies and Procedures due to Inadequate Education.

A three-year old boy is admitted to a pediatric unit following an acute asthma attack complicated by left lower lobe pneumonia. The nurse responsible for medication administration knows the boy well because the boy had been admitted to his unit several times during the past twenty-four months. During these admissions, the boy received numerous intravenous antibiotics.

As the nurse slowly pushes a syringe of Rocephin (ceftriaxone) 500mg into the child's indwelling catheter, he remembers that the child has tolerated medications better than most of his patients. The child, however, is now wearing a red "allergy alert" bracelet warning caregivers that he is allergic to ceftri-

Table 2-1. Major Medication Error Causes and Contributing Factors

Causes (first and second level categories only)

Communication
Verbal miscommunication
Written miscommunication
Misinterpretation of the order

Name Confusion
Proprietary (trade) name confusion
Established (generic) name confusion

Labeling
Immediate container labels of product—
    manufacturer, distributor or repackager
Labels of dispensed product—practitioner
Carton labeling of product—manufacturer,
    distributor or repackager
Package insert
Electronic reference material
Printed reference material
Advertising

Human Factors
Knowledge deficit
Performance deficit
Miscalculation of dosage or infusion rate
Computer error
Error in stocking/restocking/cart filling
Drug preparation error
Transcription error

Stress
Fatigue/lack of sleep
Confrontational or intimidating behavior

Packaging/Design
Inappropriate packaging or design
Dosage form (tablet/capsule) confusion
Devices

Contributing Factors: Systems Related
(first level categories only)
Lighting
Noise level
Frequent interruptions and distractions
Training
Staffing
Lack of availability of health care professional
Assignment or placement of a health care
    provider or inexperienced personnel
System for covering patient care (e.g., floating
    personnel, agency coverage)
Policies and procedures
Communication systems between health care
    practitioners
Patient counseling
Floor stock
Pre-printed medication orders
Other

Source: NCC MERP: *The NCC MERP Taxonomy of Medication Errors,* 1998. Used with permission of the Office of the Secretariat, United States Pharmacopeia.

axone/penicillin derivatives. The allergy was identified the previous month during the boy's hospital stay in another city while visiting grandparents.

The organization's medication administration policies and procedures clearly establish that a nurse must check each care recipient's name band as well as any allergy alert bands prior to any medication administration. The nurse missed one training session related to medication administration procedures, and does not know to check for the bracelet which is not visible anyway because the boy's favorite stuffed animal is wrapped around his small hand, obscuring the bracelet.

The nurse administers the medication and leaves the room with his medication cart. The boy experiences an

anaphylactic reaction to the ceftriaxone. A few minutes later, the nurse hears the screams of the boy's mother when she finds her child unresponsive.

Sentinel Event Example: Insufficient Training.
A man is admitted to a long term care facility from the orthopedic unit of a nearby hospital. The man is to receive phenytoin on a daily basis. The order reads, "(Dilantin) 400mg qd po." The unit clerk transcribes the order from the discharge order to the physician's order sheet as "phenytoin 400mg qd prn" or only as needed. Unfortunately, the pharmacy does not question this order. The medication nurse in the long term care facility is aware that the order represents an unusually high dose of phenytoin prn. However, she does not verify the order against the discharge order herself, and since the man is not experiencing seizures, no

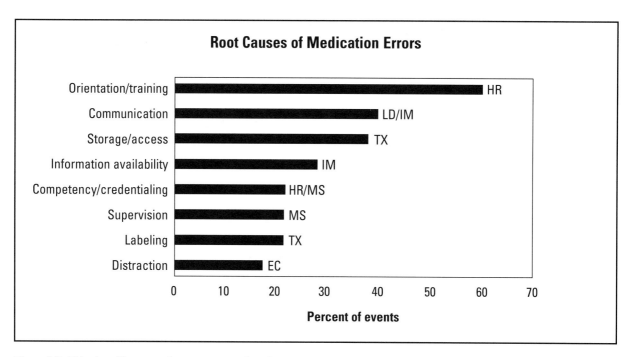

Figure 2-3. *This chart illustrates the percentage of medication errors attributed to each root cause, reported to the Joint Commission between January 1995 and January 2001.*

phenytoin is administered. On day four at the long term care facility, the night nurse during routine rounds finds the man seizing violently. He is transported to the local hospital where he is in an intensive care unit for 72 hours post admission, experiencing major seizure episodes, resulting in permanent brain damage.

Sentinel Event Example: Inadequate Education.

An 85-year old woman is admitted to the hospital for blood in the stool. Her physician schedules a colonoscopy for the following morning and writes a prescription for Ativan (lorazepam) 1.0mg to be administered 30 minutes prior to the procedure. During the past year, the hospital's nursing staff noted that lorazepam had been missing from several unit-dose drawers. Hence, the medication is now issued on a count sheet for general unit use and, since it is a controlled substance, is documented as a CII narcotic.

The nurse interprets the care recipient's dose as 10mg rather than 1.0mg since the physician had placed a terminal "0" after a decimal point. Since the physician ordered the medication to be given as soon as possible, and since the medication is maintained in narcotic floor stock, the order is not reviewed by a pharmacist prior to administration. The nurse removes ten-1mg tablets from the locked area of his

medication cart and proceeds to the care recipient's room. The alert, elderly lady questions why she is being given so many tablets. The nurse reassures her that preoperative medications are typically given in higher doses than usual.

In addition to lorazepam, the woman is receiving both furosemide and lisinopril for treatment of congestive heart failure. Both medications lower her blood pressure. When the incorrect 10mg lorazepam dose is added to these routine medications administered less than one-hour earlier, the woman suffers a cardiac arrest and dies later that afternoon.

Nursing staff orientation must ensure the staff's thorough understanding of required organization policies and procedures regarding medication administration. Supervisory staff should provide ample opportunity for a newly hired nurse to observe medication administration by an experienced nurse, using the policies and procedures approved by the organization. The new nurse's competence in this area, as observed and documented by the mentor, must be validated prior to independent medication administration by the new nurse.

Nurses must understand the critical link between complying with organization medica-

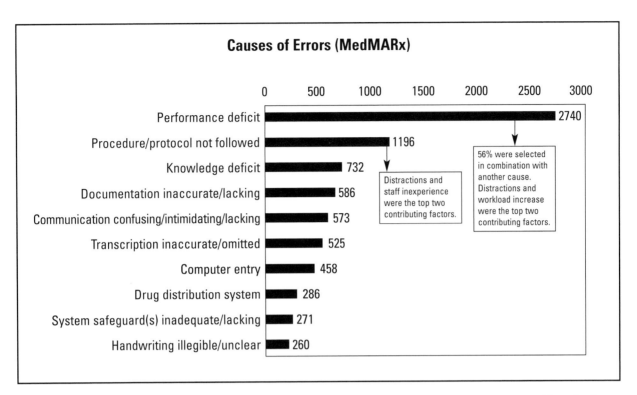

Figure 2-4. *This chart illustrates causes of errors reported to MedMarx™. It contains preliminary data abstracted from the database for the calendar year 1999.* **Source:** *U.S. Pharmacopeia. Used with permission.*

tion administration policies and procedures and safe medication administration. Giving a medication to the wrong care recipient almost always is a result of failing to follow the organization's policy for identifying the proper recipient. Administration of extra doses results from a failure to follow the organization's policy and procedures for documenting medication administration and checking the medication administration record prior to administration.

These examples illustrate the need for nurses to have a thorough understanding of important pharmacological and procedural issues surrounding medication administration, including such information as

- usual doses of frequently administered medications (for example, a usual dose of ibuprofen suspension for a twelve-month old would be 100mg every 4–6 hours, whereas a very high dose would be 300mg every 4–6 hours);

- common errors surrounding high risk medications (for example, a misplaced decimal point in a 5-FU chemotherapy order resulting in an individual receiving a one-hundred fold dose of a potent drug); and

- normal infusion rates for frequently prescribed medications (for example, 1Gm of Vancomcyin would typically be administered over two hours to avoid "red man's syndrome" resulting in the care recipient experiencing life-threatening hypotension, whereas infusing this quantity of drug over 30 minutes would reflect inadequate staff training).

Knowledge of important pharmacy issues received through training enables nurses to correlate medications, disease, and clinical status. This improves the detection of errors and promotes the detection of contraindications and adverse effects.[11]

Prevention Strategies

Request training about medications and medication administration devices. Nurses should feel comfortable about their knowledge of medications they are administering and the function and limitations of medication administration devices. If they are uncomfortable with any aspect of medication administration, they should request additional training prior to administering drugs.

Know and use time-honored techniques to reduce medication errors. One of the best safeguards against medication-related sentinel events is for nursing staff to be thoroughly trained in carefully verifying each individual's medication dose against the available clinical record. Errors frequently occur in transcription, particularly when individuals receiving care are transferred to other care settings. Nurses must reconcile individual medication containers with the medication administration record, and licensed personnel or others permitted by state law should prepare the dose.

Unit dose systems effectively reduce medication errors. Nurses should advocate for their use in all care settings. These systems eliminate multidose concentrates and the need to reconstitute medications. Drugs are stored in and administered from labeled packages of a single dose and are ready to be administered when dispensed. This enables organizations to limit floor stocks. Dosing is often the riskiest part of medication administration. One study found that 79% of administration errors in a medical intensive care unit were related to dosing.[12] One strategy to reduce dosing errors is to use dosing crib sheets that provide administration information at a glance, drug duration limits, guidelines for intramuscular versus IV administration, age-specific criteria, renal failure guidelines, neonatal/pediatric IV dosing guidelines for critically ill individuals, generic versus trade names, drug concentrations, dilutents, suggested starting dose, usual incremental changes, usual/maximal dosage range, and monitoring guidelines.

Double-checking systems effectively reduces the likelihood of errors and should be part of a nurse's training. For example, requiring two nurses to independently check the label on a unit of blood against the individual's identification band can help to reduce transfusion errors.

Root Cause 2: Communication Failure

Sentinel Event Example: Miscommunication of Information. *A 60-year old man receiving home care services complains about a headache to his home health nurse on each of the nurse's three visits during a one-week period. The man indicates that he is tired of "bothering" his primary care physician about vari-* *ous symptoms. At the conclusion of the third visit, the nurse offers to discuss the man's complaint with his primary care physician upon return to the agency. When the nurse discusses the headache with the man's physician, the physician instructs the nurse to call the local pharmacy with the following prescription:*

> *Fioricet Tabs. #30*
> *Sig: 1-2 tabs q 4-6 hours prn headache*
> *Refill x3*

In error, the nurse telephones the pharmacy and provides the following prescription:

> *Fiorinal Tabs. #30*
> *Sig: 1-2 tabs q 4-6 hours prn headache*
> *Refill x3*

The man has a long history of peptic ulcer disease, which resulted in several hospitalizations for gastrointestinal bleeding. The man began taking the Fiorinal which contains 325mg aspirin per tablet. The intended medication—Fioricet—in contrast, contains 325mg acetaminophen per tablet.

The man completes the entire first prescription and 15 tablets of the first refill. At this point, he presents to the emergency room with acute abdominal pain, blood in the stool, and a hemoglobin of 4.9. He is admitted immediately to the intensive care unit. Within hours, he needs life support. After several units of blood and a four-week hospital stay, the man recovers and is able to return to his home.

Effective communication among all health care professionals is critical to an individual's care. Illegible physician handwriting, oral orders, and order transcription account for a large percentage of drug administration errors. Fifteen percent of the medication errors reported to NCC MERP involved illegible handwriting, problems with leading and trailing zeroes, misinterpreted abbreviations, and incomplete medication orders.[13] One multidisciplinary team at a health care organization, including pharmacists, nurses, and physicians, recently studied the percentage of orders that did not include the prescriber's pager number for use with order clarification and the percentage of oral orders received.[14] The team learned that more than 20% of orders during a specified time period were received orally. Direct communication among the physician prescribing the medication, the pharmacist filling the medication, and the nurse administering the medication is rare. Since oral telephone orders are often a necessity, particularly in alternate care locations, the potential for medication errors due to miscommunication or misinterpretation is high. The shift of health care services to outpatient locations and the home setting increase the likelihood of this type of error. The opportunity for miscommunication between the individual giving the order and the clinician receiving this same order is apparent and has resulted in numerous sentinel events throughout the health care field.

Prevention Strategies

Ask questions. As an educated and valuable member of the health care team, the nurse should feel comfortable in questioning both physicians and pharmacists regarding choice of medications, administration routes, dosages, interactions, and reactions. Nurses should question all those involved to resolve each of his or her concerns prior to medication administration.

Clarify orders. All too often, nurses struggle to decipher illegible handwriting and to complete incomplete orders. Prior to medication administration, nurses should ensure that all orders are clarified and complete. The NCC MERP recommends that any order that is incomplete, illegible, or of any other concern should be clarified prior to administration using an established process for resolving questions.[15] Nurses should comply with organization policies regarding verbal order safeguards, such as the nurse reading telephone orders back to the ordering provider, or repeating or spelling any drug names or dosages. Order clarification is particularly critical in settings where pharmacists do not have an opportunity to review the physician order. For example, nurses in long term care, behavioral health care, and home care organizations frequently communicate physician orders over the telephone to pharmacists in a different location. Sending legible orders via facsimile machine can help reduce the likelihood of error and get the prescription into the nurse's hands more quickly. Some organizations use e-mail to transmit physician orders, which

requires that the order by typed. Illegible handwriting is not an issue. When orders are sent via fax or e-mail, nurses and administrative staff should take extra care that the information is kept confidential.

Take extra precaution with error-prone medications through increased communication. The professional literature is full of reports of medications known to have been involved frequently with serious medication errors. According to the ISMP, the five high-alert medications are insulin, opiates and narcotics, injectable potassium chloride (or phosphate) concentrate, intravenous anticoagulants (heparin), and sodium chloride solutions above 0.9 percent.[16] For example, use of "trailing zeroes" with insulin leads to inappropriate administration. An order for Humulin Insulin NPH, written as "10.0 Units" SQ AM and PM, can very easily be misinterpreted by the pharmacist and nurse as "100 Units" SQ AM and PM. Therefore, physicians and other prescribers should *never* write insulin orders with a trailing zero. When there is a trailing zero, the nurse must clarify the order prior to administration. This extra communication is critical. Other risk factors associated with high-alert medications and error-reduction strategies that nurses either can implement or participate in system-wide implementation appear as Table 2-2, page 26.

Communicate with and educate the individual receiving the medication. Nurses should identify for the care recipient and family, as appropriate, each medication he or she is administering at the time of administration. If a new medication is being given, the nurse should take time to educate the individual and family about the medication and provide available literature describing the drug and side effects that may be experienced. Communication and education in any care setting help to reduce the likelihood that an individual at a later date will receive the incorrect medication, a medication intended for another person, or that a dose will be omitted.

In addition, an individual with adequate information about a medication that he or she is allergic to will be better able to help prevent future allergic reactions. The individual receiving care must be an active partner in the

Table 2-2. High-Alert Medication Safety: Risk Factors and Suggested Error-Reduction Strategies

Insulin
Common Risk Factors
- Lack of dose check systems
- Insulin and heparin vials kept in close proximity to each other on a nursing unit, leading to mix-ups
- Use of "U" as an abbreviation for "units" in orders (which can be confused with "O," resulting in a 10-fold overdose)
- Incorrect rates being programmed into an infusion pump

Suggested Strategies
- Establish a check system whereby one nurse prepares the dose and another nurse reviews it.
- Do not store insulin and heparin near each other.
- Build in an independent check system for infusion pump rates and concentration settings.

Opiates and Narcotics
Common Risk Factors
- Parenteral narcotics stored in nursing areas as floor stock
- Confusion between hydromorphone and morphine
- Patient-controlled analgesia (PCA) errors regarding concentration and rate

Suggested Strategies
- Limit the opiates and narcotics available in floor stock.
- Educate staff about hydromorphone and morphine mix-ups.
- Implement PCA protocols that include double-checks of the drug, pump setting, and dosage.

Injectable Potassium Chloride or Phosphate Concentrate
Common Risk Factors
- Storing concentrated potassium chloride/ phosphate outside of the pharmacy

- Mixing potassium chloride/phosphate extemporaneously
- Requests for unusual concentrations

Suggested Strategies
- Remove potassium chloride/phosphate from floor stock.
- Move drug preparation off units and use commercially available premixed IV solutions.
- Standardize and limit drug concentrations.

Intravenous Anticoagulants (Heparin)
Common Risk Factors
- Unclear labeling regarding concentration and total volume
- Multi-dose containers
- Confusion between heparin and insulin due to similar measurement units and proximity

Suggested Strategies
- Standardize concentrations and use premixed solutions.
- Use only single-dose containers.
- Separate heparin and insulin and remove heparin from the top of medication carts.

Sodium Chloride Solutions above 0.9 percent
Common Risk Factors
- Storing sodium chloride solutions (above 0.9 percent) on nursing units
- Large number of concentrations/formulations available
- No double-check system in place

Suggested Strategies
- Limit access of sodium chloride solutions (above 0.9 percent) and remove from nursing units.
- Standardize and limit drug concentrations.
- Double-check pump rate, drug, concentration and line attachments.

Source: Joint Commission: High-alert medications and patient safety. *Sentinel Event Alert,* Issue 11, November, 1999.

medication use process and should be encouraged to ask questions and express concerns. Compliance is often a key issue. As with physicians and pharmacists who interact with care recipients, nurses should stress as part of the education process the importance of the individual's responsibility regarding medication use. The NCC MERP recommends that at the time of administration, the name, purpose, and effects of each medication be discussed with the care recipient and/or caregiver.[15]

Root Cause 3: Failure to Ensure Safe Medication Storage/Access

"Near Miss" Example: Unsafe Medication and Equipment Storage. *A 72-year old man is admitted to a long term care facility following surgery with a diagnosis of carcinoma of the colon with metastatic disease. He receives total parenteral nutrition (TPN) with electrolytes, trace elements, insulin, and lipids as his sole nutrition source. A central line is in place for the infusion. After receiving TPN for two weeks, he develops an infection involving the methicillin-resistant staph aureus organism. His physician orders Vancomycin to combat the infection. The nursing home staff administers both the TPN and Vancomycin via infusion pumps. While the man is receiving both, his physician also decides to try an experimental antineoplastic agent to combat the carcinoma. At the same time, the man experiences severe pain that necessitates intravenous morphine via analgesic infusion pump.*

One evening, as a nurse is preparing to administer the man's infusion, she notices that his morphine cassettes and experimental drug are missing from the refrigerator in the medication room. In addition, she discovers that the refrigerator appears to be malfunctioning because the TPN and Vancomycin solutions are warm. The facility had not placed a lock on the refrigerator door and the nurse kept the medication room unlocked so that nursing aides could obtain with ease enteral nutrition stored in the room. In addition, the morphine pump is missing, and the parenteral nutrition pump and pump used to infuse Vancomycin are not plugged into an electrical outlet to recharge their batteries.

The nurse immediately calls the administrator for assistance. The administrator contacts the pharmacy to obtain the necessary medications for the man.

Fortunately, the pharmacy is able to respond in an urgent manner, providing the medications and two fully-charged pumps within two hours. Had this not happened, the man could have suffered serious adverse effects as a result of the delay.

Sentinel Event Example: Unsafe Medication Storage. *A 78-year old woman residing in a behavioral health facility frequently attempts to take items from the top of medication carts. In the past, she has taken a nurse's soda can and examination gloves used to empty medication bottles.*

Unfortunately, while returning to the nurses' station to answer a telephone call, a nurse leaves his cart unattended. On top of the cart is an open and almost full bottle of povidone iodine. The 78-year old woman removes the bottle of povidone solution from the cart top and drinks the entire amount. She is rushed via ambulance to the local hospital emergency room where emergency staff take measures to neutralize the ingestion. Unfortunately, the woman sustains damage to her esophagus, which results in her being unable to take nutrition orally for the rest of her life.

The first example illustrates organizational problems with equipment management, monitoring the drug storage environment, staff education, and security. The long term care facility failed to keep equipment in a ready mode for infusion and failed to monitor the temperature of the refrigerator used to store medications. In addition, the staff was not sufficiently educated regarding security and storage of medications, and the facility did not ensure appropriate security for controlled substances.

Wandering care recipients in any health care setting, not just behavioral, may drink an unsecured item that is intended for external use only. The second example illustrates the importance of ensuring medication security.

Prevention Strategies

Ensure proper implementation of organization's medication storage policies and procedures. Although pharmacists most often are responsible for establishing medication storage policies and procedures, the nursing staff should help ensure that the policies and procedures are followed at all times. Nurses must secure a medication cart whenever it is unattended, even for a few moments, and make certain that medications are not left unsecured in open areas, for example, on top of medication carts, on the counter at the nursing station, or on tables in eating/feeding areas while other individuals are receiving care.

Guard against medication theft. Nurses have a responsibility to guard against medication theft, particularly in units where medications are kept at the bedside. Storage at the bedside provides convenience in medication administration and while training individuals for self-administration during transition to home or assisted-living settings.

However, such storage also brings with it additional responsibility to guard against theft by both individuals receiving care and visitors. In all cases, medications must be secured. A nurse on each shift must determine whether or not proper security has been maintained. Emergency medications must be controlled and secured in care areas. Nurses can help ensure that crash carts are adequately stocked and secured. A lack of either can lead to a serious adverse drug event.

Minimize after-hours access to the pharmacy. According to the ASHP,

> Routine access to the pharmacy after hours by nonpharmacists (for example, nurses) to obtain medications is strongly discouraged. This practice should certainly be minimized to the fullest extent possible. The available medications should be limited to those most often needed for immediate administration after hours and policies and procedures clearly understood by this group of nurses, should be readily available. In addition, new orders for any high risk medications, should be reviewed by an on-call pharmacist prior to administration. The drugs in this designated "after-hours" area should be available in the most ready form possible (for example, unit dose).[17]

On-site pharmacy services are often available to nurses working in acute care settings 24 hours per day, 7 days per week. However, smaller organizations may not be able to provide such access. Long term care organizations typically use portable emergency boxes or night cabinets for after-hours access and allow access by order only. A health care organization with limited pharmacy hours could also design a system whereby a nurse in need for pharmacy assistance could contact another organization with 24-hour pharmacy hours.

Evaluate with pharmacists the need for floor stocks and reduce or eliminate these whenever possible. Floor stock needs should be evaluated on an ongoing basis by representatives of nursing and pharmacy. Such stocks can create a serious potential for medication errors and adverse effects in all types of health care organizations. Floor stock is frequently used without having ensured a proper medication assessment by a pharmacist. This can result in serious clinical medication errors. For example, if an individual receives regular high doses of acetaminophen tablets from floor stock and the pharmacy dispenses routine doses of propoxyphene/APAP, serious complications could arise for the individual, potentially resulting in liver toxicity. Such potential must be considered for every medication allowed as floor stock. The use of multiple cabinets of floor stock runs the risk of inadequate accountability for the "mini pharmacies." Floor stock medications generally should be limited to those for emergency use and routinely used safe items, such as mouthwash and antiseptic solutions.

Keeping floor stock to an absolute minimum and withdrawing dangerous products will decrease the likelihood of medication errors. Dangerous floor stock items such as concentrated potassium chloride and other concentrated solutions need to be eliminated. Following sentinel events involving concentrated potassium chloride (KCl), the Joint Commission issued a *Sentinel Event Alert* in 1998 making the health care community aware of the serious potential for sentinel events with this drug.[18] Storage of concentrated KCl directly adjacent to other similar looking vials, such as sterile water for injection or bacteriostatic sodium chloride, can lead to improper medication selection. This, in turn, can lead to sentinel events such as severe cardiac rhythm disturbances and death when nurses inadvertently give concentrated KCl IV push instead of the other solutions.

Root Cause 4: Insufficient Information Availability

Sentinel Event Example: Lack of Critical Information. *An 88-year old woman with a history of recent hospitalization for esophageal disease is admitted to the Alzheimer's unit of a small long term care facility. She brings with her a 90-day supply of numerous medications. Her family arranges with the facility's administrator to use this supply before ordering medications from the organization's pharmacy provider. One of her daily medications is Alendronate sodium (Fosamax), used for the treatment of osteoporosis. The nurse on the unit is new and not familiar with Fosamax. She consults the most recent edition of a drug reference book available at the nursing station. Unfortunately, the resource is very dated and does not include information on Fosamax. The nurse consults with another new colleague who indicates that his mother had experienced some stomach upset while on the medication. The woman's nurse decides to administer the drug just prior to bedtime since she hopes this could help to reduce stomach upset.*

Unfortunately, product literature on Fosamax indicates that the drug must be given on an empty stomach, with a full glass of water, to an individual who is upright and must remain in this position for 30 minutes after receiving the drug and until the first meal of the day has been eaten.

Within 14 days, the woman is admitted to an area emergency room with weight loss, bloody emesis, and blood in the stool. She is placed on total parenteral nutrition therapy, but dies six days later.

Nurses who administer medications must have easy access to current drug information as close to the point of use as possible. This could include the organization's formulary, a current nursing drug reference book, and a current copy of *Physicians Desk Reference* (this also can be accessed online at www.pdr.net). Such references provide the nurse with indications for medications, expected outcomes, potential adverse events, and appropriate actions to take if adverse events occur.

In addition, all persons who administer medications need to have adequate access to information on the care recipient as close to the administration point as possible. Key information includes medical history, reported allergies, and prognosis and treatment plan. This infor-

mation allows the nurse to assess the appropriateness of administering a particular medication to a particular individual. An incomplete, unavailable, or inaccurate history and physical and nursing assessment, including a medication history, can lead to prescribing and administering a drug to which the individual is allergic or to adverse drug interactions.

Prevention Strategies

Ensure access to reliable and current drug information. As mentioned earlier, nurses should ask questions about drugs with which they are unfamiliar. Pharmacists are the medication experts and should be consulted to answer nurses' questions. If a medication is too new to be described in published reference sources, nurses must receive appropriate information. "As pharmacology and technology advances, patients should be able to expect a nurse who is continually updated on new medications and the ways they are delivered," noted one nurse during public testimony on medication error prevention strategies.[19] "Good nursing practice dictates that nurses are never to administer a drug they are unfamiliar with. If an individual is to receive a drug that is too new to be in the usual reference books, nurses should insist that information be provided to them. And they should not administer that drug until they have enough information to be comfortable doing so."[19] An organization's pharmacy may facilitate the availability of drug information by posting or otherwise providing drug alerts, including specific precautions for medications.

Ensure timely access to appropriate information on the individual receiving care. Again, nurses must have timely access to critical information on the care recipient in order to assess the appropriateness of medications. Identification of medications requiring immediate dosing or medications that could be delayed will also assist in acquiring accurate, timely information.

Root Cause 5: Inadequate Competence Assessment and Credentialing

"Near Miss" Example: Inadequate Competence Assessment. *A 16-year old boy is admitted to home health care after discharge from same-day surgery where he had his left anterior cruciate ligament (ACL)*

repaired following a basketball injury. The surgery center's discharging nurse had connected the youth to an ambulatory infusion pump so that he could receive a continuous morphine infusion during the next three days. The order read: "Morphine Sulfate 2mg/hour continuous with a 0.5mg bolus every 10 minutes up to 4/hour."

Although the discharging nurse had not previously used this ambulatory device, she made the comment, "How hard can this be to connect? All of these things work exactly the same." The day surgery nurse set the pump to deliver 20mg per hour instead of 2mg per hour as ordered.

When the home health nurse arrived at the youth's home at 9:00 PM that evening for an admission visit, the parents immediately expressed concern, asked about their son's unresponsiveness, and about whether this was normal with pain medication. The youth had been receiving 20mg per hour for the last eight hours. He had respirations of 4 and a blood pressure of 70/40.

The home health nurse immediately telephoned 911. Upon arrival at the local emergency room, the boy was intubated and placed on a respirator. Fortunately, he left the hospital four days later with no apparent problems.

Numerous medication-related errors have been traced to an organization's failure to validate competence or require special credentials to care for particular individuals with special needs. The nurse in this example had not been deemed competent in the use of a new type of pump. An organization must define what competencies are to be assessed, frequency of assessment, method of assessment, and who, by education and training, is qualified to assess specified competence.

Prevention Strategies

Ensure ability to meet performance expectations stated in job descriptions. Every accredited health care organization is expected to assess each staff member's ability to meet required performance expectations. Competence of all involved in the medication use process is critical to its optimal performance and prevention of sentinel events. Lack of competence anywhere along the process can increase the probability of a med-

ication error. "Evaluation of one's performance by peers is a hallmark of professionalism and a method by which the profession is held accountable to society. Nurses must be willing to have their practice reviewed and evaluated by their peers," notes ANA's *Code for Nurses.*[20]

Assume personal responsibility for competence. According to the ANA's *Code for Nurses,* the profession of nursing is obligated to provide adequate and competent nursing care. "Therefore, it is the personal responsibility of each nurse to maintain competency in practice," notes the *Code for Nurses.* "For the client's optimum well-being and for the nurse's own professional development, the care of the client reflects and incorporates new techniques and knowledge in health care as these develop, especially as they relate to the nurse's particular field of practice. The nurse . . . must assume personal responsibility for currency of knowledge and skills."[20]

Use information to identify potential for sentinel events. Be informed. Circulate relevant materials to nurse colleagues. Nurses should increase their awareness of the types of medication errors occurring, risk factors, root causes, and prevention strategies. Regularly reading professional literature such as the Joint Commission's *Sentinel Event Alert* (*www.jcaho.org*), and organization newsletters and performance improvement results, and attending inservice education can decrease the possibility of sentinel events due to medication errors.

Root Cause 6: Labeling Error

Sentinel Event Example: Labeling Error. *A 60-year old man recovering from hip replacement surgery is admitted to a nursing facility. His physician orders atenolol (Tenormin) 100mg qd (that is, daily) for hypertension. A pharmacist at the pharmacy used by the facility enters the order into the computer system in error, as atenolol 100mg q.i.d. (that is, four times a day).*

Since the normal dose of the medication is 50–100mg daily, this labeling error leads to the administration of an extremely high dose of this medication. The man receives the high dose for a 96-hour period. On day four, during morning rounds, a day nurse finds the man completely unresponsive. The man is resuscitated, transported to the local emergency room, and placed on a respirator. He suffers permanent brain damage.

A properly labeled medication allows the nurse to perform a key function that ensures medication administration accuracy. The nurse asks, "Is the medication about to be administered the right medication? Is it in the right dose? Is it for the right individual? Is it to be administered by the right route? Is it being given at the right time?" Although labeling errors are initiated in the pharmacy, they can be caught by a well-trained, competent nurse prior to medication administration, thereby reducing the likelihood of sentinel events.

Prevention Strategy

Administer only properly labeled medications and check the label three times. According to NCC MERP, any person administering medication to an individual should administer only medications that are properly labeled. During the administration process, the nurse should read the label three times to ensure accuracy. Reading should occur when 1) the medication is prepared or reached for, 2) immediately prior to administering the medication, and 3) when discarding the container or placing it into the storage location.[15]

Root Cause 7: Unsafe Environment of Care

Imagine a nursing area that is poorly lit, crowded and cluttered with loose papers, medication carts, chairs, and desks. Multiple conversations are occurring simultaneously. Distractions abound. In this environment, a nurse is trying to draw up doses for several individuals. She is interrupted while preparing the medication, accidentally switching one person's medications with another's. Amidst such chaos, it is easy to understand how a wrong drug or dose might be drawn up and administered or how an incorrect dosage might be noted in an individual's medication administration record.

Health care leaders must ensure that the environment has appropriate space and equipment for preparing medication dosages. Providing an efficient work environment can prevent medica-tion administration errors. Nurses, like many other health care professionals, function better in well-lit, clean, and quiet work spaces. Organizations serious about preventing medication use errors are aware of the role played by the physical workplace, and ensure that the workplace has the appropriate space and equipment. Factors such as lighting, temperature control, noise-level, and distractions, such as telephones or the performance of unrelated tasks, should be examined.[15]

Prevention Strategy

Take the time and find the space to stop and think. Distractions abound in all health care environments. As staffing shortages and care recipient acuity increase, nurses are stretched thinner and thinner. "But we are human, we are all fallible. There is only so much sensory input a person can handle, only so many questions we can process at a time. When we find our minds so overloaded that we are unable to think, we have the right to stop and do so," notes one nurse administrator and educator.[19] Nurses must take the time to think about the care they are providing.

Communicate inappropriate environmental condition to the appropriate parties. If a nurse feels the organization's environment is not conducive to safe and accurate preparation of medications it is his or her responsibility to report this concern to the director of nursing or environmental staff, as appropriate. The nurse should provide specific information on why current conditions are unsafe or otherwise inappropriate, identify what type of conditions are needed, and offer suggestions on how the present environment could be improved.

Technology and Error Prevention

Health care leaders should be aware of the technology available to assist nurses in the prevention of medication errors. Whenever possible, computerization and automation of error-prone steps in the medication administration system can provide a key risk reduction tool. Key systems widely available today include computerized medication administration records, computerized physician order entry systems, automated dispensing units, bar coding technology, and automated infusion pumps. A description of each follows.

Computerized Medication Administration Records

Computerized medication administration records (MARs) have greatly reduced medication errors, particularly those related to transcription. One document is shared between pharmacy, the point of dispensing, and nursing, the point of administration. This precludes the need for two sets of manual records that must be accurate and updated as each medication change occurs. One manual record drives dispensing and clinical review by pharmacists and the other, "a kardex," directs administration and recording of medications by nurses.[21] Data elements in manual systems often differ, and errors can occur when changes in the dispensing record are not reflected in the administration record. Transcription errors, frequently occurring as orders are entered in the MAR, account for a very large proportion of all medication errors. Transition to a computerized MAR in all health care settings can reduce errors involving legibility of orders. The use of a shared medication record by pharmacy and nursing can improve efficiency, speed delivery of medications and information, and decrease the likelihood of medication errors.

Computerized Physician Order Entry Systems

Similarly, computerized physician order entry (CPOE) systems can reduce medication errors at the ordering and prescribing stages, earlier in the medication use system. CPOE or "electronic prescribing" is capable of eliminating many problems associated with prescribing. With electronic prescribing, a physician, while in his or her office or examination room, uses a computer or hand-held electronic device to generate a prescription and electronically transfer the order to the pharmacy. Available systems can check a drug's indication against a diagnosis, warn of allergies and drug interactions, review lab tests, flag potential problems, display a menu of acceptable doses, suggest optimal doses, refuse to accept an order until the prescriber chooses the dose, route, and dosing

schedule, eliminate reliance on handwritten and verbal orders, and suggest less expensive but equally effective medications.

However, organizations need to exercise caution in ensuring that the CPOE systems they select and implement properly interface with the pharmacy's computerized systems. Some "stand-alone" CPOE systems available in the marketplace allow physicians to enter data while on the unit, in their offices, and so forth, but do not directly interface with the organization's pharmacy system. This means that, although the physician order is neatly transcribed by the computer, the staff is not able to receive information such as allergy warnings, drug interactions warnings, or dose range checking available through the pharmacy computerized system. Initial medication doses must be reviewed by pharmacy staff before administered by nurses. When properly designed and implemented, CPOE systems do add another layer of checks and balances to the medication use process, making it less likely for errors to occur.

Automated Dispensing Units

Automated dispensing units (ADUs) can decrease medication administration errors if used properly. Nurses indicate that, with ADUs, they spend less time searching for missing doses and waiting for doses to arrive from the pharmacy. Both factors have been associated with errors of omission. ADUs are frequently used in acute care settings to control floor stock, control and improve accountability for narcotic use, or control and improve accountability for the use of emergency or first-dose medications after pharmacy hours.

The early systems replaced the need for a nursing supervisor to enter the pharmacy after hours or dispense from a nursing unit "night cupboard." Early prototypes used an automated unit dose dispensing machine at each care recipient's bedside. Others now allow medications to be placed on nursing units in a controlled environment in advance of physician orders. Security is ensured through electronic passwords or other means that identify the person removing the medication and the individual for whom the dose is intended. Still others make extensive use of state-of-the-art computer software, robotics, and bar coding technology throughout the medication distribution system. Following proper user identification, many systems currently allow the nurse to open only the drawer in which the correct medication is stored (or the drawer opens automatically), thus eliminating the number of medications from which to select and decreasing the chance for error.

Studies published in scientific literature focus on automated dispensing systems and their relationship to medication errors. One organization indicated that after implementing an automated system, medication errors steadily decreased even though the total number of doses administered to care recipients actually increased by 15%.[22] Such systems are not fail safe, however, and have been associated with medication errors. One expert outlined how automated systems can and do fail, maintaining that, "Excessive faith in technological solutions and in the infallibility of such systems has often left users unprepared for the consequences of system failure."[23]

Too heavy a reliance on technology creates different problems. Some report that nurses appear to do less checking when relying on automated systems. Thus, doses the nurses would have checked if they had taken them out of a cart drawer were not checked because of reliance on the machine. Or, a nurse could retrieve a drug from an automated dispenser before a pharmacist screens the order for allergies or double-checks the dose, thereby circumventing the usual checks and balances between pharmacists and nurses. If a sleeve that dispenses doses of a specific medication is filled with the wrong medication, several doses may be administered before the error is discovered. Moreover, some automated dispensers are poorly designed, allowing a medication to drop into the wrong slot. Or, they may be stocked haphazardly, allowing adult and pediatric strengths of a medication to be placed next to each other.[24]

The Joint Commission requires that proper medication control systems, designed to prevent medication errors, are in place when automated dispensing devices are used.[25] An important element of a thorough control system is pharmacist review of all prescriptions or orders. This element must not be bypassed with ADU systems. A blended system often works best to reduce administration errors. The pharmacist releases the majority of medications after entry or review. However, medications that are required immediately, such as opiates for pain control, can have an "override" function that allows a dose to be released to the registered nurse. This is similar to narcotics maintained on floor stocks in a manual system. Discrepancy reports generated in the pharmacy indicate medications dispensed without an order confirmed by a pharmacist. Reconciliation of the discrepancy reports according to time frames defined by organization policy closes the loop on systems monitoring. Most ADU systems also will generate a report indicating the staff members who use the override feature more frequently than others in comparable roles.

When an emergency need for a drug does not allow time for the pharmacist review prior to dispensing, the Joint Commission permits emergency dispensing from ADUs when significant harm to the individual receiving care could result from the delay involved for a pharmacist review of the medication order. If the medication involved will be provided on an ongoing basis following the first dose, the Joint Commission expects the order to be sent to the pharmacy and reviewed by the pharmacist before the next dose of drug is administered.

Organizations should consider the legal issues associated with the use of ADUs. The attorney general in one state recently ruled that the use of ADUs in nursing homes violates state pharmacy laws, which require facilities that dispense prescription medications to be under a pharmacist's continuous on-site supervision. Explains Darryl Rich, PharmD, of the Joint Commission, "Many pharmacy boards are determining that unlimited nursing access to these automated dispensing devices without a pharmacist review and 'release of the drug for removal from the machine' is considered the act of 'dispensing,' which nurses are not allowed to do under most state nursing practice acts, even in hospitals."[25] Hence, prior to using ADUs, leaders from the organization must ensure the organization's compliance with state legal and regulatory requirements.

Bar Coding Technology

Bar coding technology combined with either robotics or ADUs is perhaps the most sophisticated technology currently used for medication administration control. The individual receiving care is assigned a bar code upon admission. All medications have a specific bar code. Each staff member administering medications has a scanner. The MAR for the individual receiving care is scanned, the dose is scanned, and the individual's wristband is scanned. The scanner sounds an alarm if the individual, drug, and order do not match. Administration errors and near misses related to wrong person, wrong drug, wrong dose, wrong route, and wrong time can be averted. Averted errors can be tracked and trended. The sole issue for many health care organizations is cost.

Constant vigilance is required in monitoring the use of bar coding systems and ensuring nurse training about their benefits and proper use. Many organizations that have implemented such systems report that nurses bypass the system by cutting the bar code off the individual's wrist and placing it in the medication bin. They then scan the product and individual's wrist band at the medication cart to save time and reduce effort. This practice eliminates all of the system's error-reduction benefits. Clearly, nursing support for bar coding systems is critical.

Infusion Devices

High-tech infusion devices warrant consideration and support by nurses due to their ability to reduce medication administration errors. Infusion pumps have definitely assisted the nurse in the administration of medications which must be delivered intravenously. For ambulatory care recipients and individuals receiving care at home, infusion pumps can deliver large doses at timed intervals. Such pumps usually are more timely and accurate than manual dosing. However, the devices are accurate only if they have been programmed accurately and are operated accurately. To avoid

errors of omission, under and over dosing, personnel must be trained in their use and assessed regularly. Control functions, safety features, and programming requirements frequently differ by pump. Hence, because all pumps are not the same, staff must receive training specific to the pump(s) they will be using.

The first potential for error is the inaccurate entering of either the flow rate or dose. Working together, nurses and pharmacists can reduce errors in this area by having pharmacists program the device and then nurses validate the program at the point of administration. If pharmacy is unable to provide this service, many organizations require two nurses to validate that the appropriate administration information has been programmed into the device prior to delivery to the care recipient. This is particularly important when high risk medications such as pain management drugs and chemotherapy agents are being delivered via the pump.

In addition, individuals receiving care and their families must be educated. Care recipients and their families need to be taught how to handle pump alarms, how to check reservoir volumes, and when to call for assistance. Alarms that are not loud enough to awaken an individual or a family member in the case of a comatose or pediatric care recipient are associated with dosing errors. A dose cannot flow into an individual if he or she is crimping the tubing while sleeping on it. If the individual does not hear the alarm and correct the problem, the dose will not be administered. Health care organizations must ensure that infusion devices are tested between use and receive preventive maintenance according to manufacturers' recommendations.

In the acute care setting and in home care, patient-controlled analgesia (PCA) often involves an infusion device for pain control. Once again, the utility of the PCA pump is dependent on programmer and operator accuracy and ability. Each individual's response is unique. The nurse and pharmacist must educate the care recipient about the use of the device and the importance of controlling pain in the healing process. The care team is responsible for assessing the response, determining the effective dose to relieve pain, and ensuring that the correct dose is delivered. If the unit is programmed correctly but the individual in pain is not able to push the button to deliver a dose, correct administration cannot occur. Frequent assessment is necessary since the need for pain management medication can change quickly, for example, when a care recipient ambulates, receives physical therapy, or increases current activity level.

Although infusion devices have decreased errors in medication administration overall, improper use of otherwise safe devices and use of unsafe devices have been highlighted by the press during the past year. According to the first of a three-part article appearing in the September 11, 2000 issue of the *Chicago Tribune,* since 1995, 39 care recipients have received fatal overdoses and 373 others have been injured while using infusion pumps capable of delivering rapid, uncontrolled bursts of medication.[26] A number of infusion devices on the market have been associated with deaths due to malfunction. Some infusion pumps prevent free-flow, a condition in which the entire contents of the intravenous solution are rapidly administered to the individual (for example, 3 liters in 10 minutes); others do not have this safety feature. Certain patient-controlled analgesic pumps also have been associated with medication administration errors due to design flaws.

In November 2000, the Joint Commission issued a *Sentinel Event Alert* warning the health care community of the potentially fatal problems associated with the use of infusion devices.[27] Experts cited indicated that the use only of infusion pumps that require set-based free-flow protection could eliminate many serious situations. Unfortunately, even many of the devices with such protection may be problematic if either the nurse administering the medication or a staff member of the agency or company providing the device deactivates or bypasses the flow rate protection. For example, "dummy clips" are being used to replace or bypass flow rate protectors and alarms are deactivated so that flow rate protectors are not effective. Both practices increase the likelihood of serious adverse events. Many other devices require the nurse to attach an in-line flow rate protection system of some kind.

When staff training or staffing is inadequate and care load increases, omission of this step can occur, thereby compromising an individual's safety. For example, a care recipient's tubing is removed from the infusion device to perform a function such as taking the individual to another department for a procedure. The built-in safety mechanism to automatically clamp off the tubing if the nurse should forget to close the roller clamp has been bypassed, thereby placing the individual in jeopardy.

Nursing staff should always make certain that the pump is being used as the manufacturer intended, with all safety features engaged. NCC MERP recommends use of only those devices that prevent free-flow.[15] In addition, nursing administration should insist on the use of only a limited number of infusion devices in order to ensure that coordinated education occurs and all staff are knowledgeable about the safety features of the devices being used. Nurses play a key role in the selection of appropriate infusion devices to be used by the organization. Consideration of safety features should be one of the key criteria in selection and purchase decisions.

Closing Comments

As a key player in the medication use process, nurses can proactively help to prevent medication errors. Proper training and competence assessment ensure that nurses are knowledgeable about medication administration and error reduction techniques. Enhanced communication among nurses, pharmacists, prescribers, and care recipients and their families can prevent errors at various stages of the medication use process. Nurses can help to ensure safe medication storage and access and the proactive elimination of medications with serious potential for adverse effects from floor stocks. Reliable and timely access to current drug information and information on the care recipient can help nurses catch potentially serious medication errors. Technological innovations such as automated dispensing units, computerized physician order entry systems, bar coding, and infusion devices can help to prevent medication errors. Nurses and other health care team members must do their part to ensure proper use.

References

1. Nadzam DM: A systems approach to medication use. In Cousins DD (ed): *Medication Use: A Systems Approach to Reducing Errors.* Oakbrook Terrace, IL: Joint Commission, 1998.

2. Leape LL, et al: Systems analysis of adverse drug events. *JAMA* 274:35–43, 1995.

3. National Coordinating Council for Medication Error Reporting and Prevention: About medication errors, 1998–99. Web site: *www.nccmerp.org/ aboutmederrors.htm.*

4. Bates DW, et al: Incidence of adverse drug events and potential adverse drug events. *JAMA* 274(1): 29–34, 1995.

5. American Society of Health-System Pharmacists: Suggested definitions and relationships among medication misadventures, medication errors, adverse drug events, and adverse drug reactions, Jan 15, 1998. Web site: *www.ashp.com/public/ proad/mederror/draftdefin.html.*

6. American Society of Health-System Pharmacists: Survey of top patient concerns: Research report, September 1999. ASHP Online: *www.ashp.org/ public/proad/hsp_week/ cons_out.html.*

7. National Patient Safety Foundation at the American Medical Association: *Public Opinion of Patient Safety Issues: Research Findings.* Sep 1997. Web site: *www.npsf.org.*

8. Bates DW, et al: Incidence of adverse drug events and potential adverse drug events. *JAMA* 274(1): 29–34, 1995.

9. Berwick DM, et al: Reducing adverse drug events and medical errors. Presented at the National Forum on Quality Improvement in Health Care Conference, New Orleans: Dec 4–7, 1996.

10. Phillips DP, Christenfeld N, Glynn LM: Increase in U.S. medication-error deaths between 1983 and 1993. *Lancet* 351:643–644, 1998.

11. Pepper GA: Errors in drug administration by nurses. *Am J Health-Syst Pharm* 52:390–395, 1995.

12. Tissot E, et al: Medication errors at the administration stage in an intensive care unit. *Intensive Care Medicine* 25:353–359, 1999.

13. National Coordinating Council for Medication Error Reporting and Prevention: Council identifies and makes recommendations to improve error-prone aspects of prescription writing. Rockville, MD: United States Pharmacopeial Convention; 4 Sep 1996, as referenced in *Am J Health-Syst Pharm* 57:Suppl 4, p S19, Dec 15, 2000.

14. Meyer TA: Improving the quality of the order-writing process for inpatient orders and outpatient prescriptions. *Am J of Health-Syst Pharm* 57: Suppl, p S19, Dec 15, 2000.

15. National Coordinating Council for Medication Error Reporting and Prevention: Recommendations to reduce errors related to administration of drugs. Rockville, MD: United States Pharmacopeial Convention; adopted Jun 29, 1999.

16. Cohen MR, Kilo CM: High-alert medications: Safeguarding against errors. In Cohen MR (ed): *Medication Errors.* Washington, DC: American Pharmaceutical Association, 1999, pp 5.1–5.40.

17. American Society of Health-System Pharmacists: *Practice Standards of ASHP* (1996–1997). ASHP guidelines: minimum standard for pharmacies in hospitals, and ASHP technical assistance bulletin on hospital drug distribution and control, pp 34, 101.

18. Joint Commission: Medication error prevention— Potassium chloride. *Sentinel Event Alert* Issue 1, Feb 27, 1998.

19. Cook MC: Nurses' six rights for safe medication administration: Testimony on behalf of the Massachusetts Nurses Association Congress on Nursing Practice before the Joint Committee on Health Care, Jun 1999. Web site: *www.massnurses.org/news/newsarchive.htm.*

20. American Nurses Association (ANA): *Code for Nurses with Interpretive Statements.* Washington, DC: ANA, 1985. (Code under review as of press date.)

21. Wilson AL, et al: Computerized medication administration records decrease medication occurrences. *Pharm Pract Manager Q* 17(1):17–29, 1997.

22. Pyxis Web Site: Success stories: Johns Hopkins, Mar 2000. Web site: *www.pyxis.com/html/success/index.asp.*

23. Tribble DA: How automated systems can (and do) fail. *Am J Hosp Pharm* 53:2622–2627, 1996.

24. Cohen MR, Cohen HG: Medication errors: Following a game plan. *Nursing* 96, Nov 1996, Web site: *www.springnet.com.*

25. Rich D: Ask the Joint Commission: Automated dispensing devices. *Hosp Pharm,* Jun 2000.

26. A three-part series by Michael J. Berens published by the *Chicago Tribune* on Sep 10–12, 2000.

27. Joint Commission: Infusion pumps: Preventing future adverse events. *Sentinel Event Alert* Issue 15, Nov 30, 2000.

Chapter 3:

Preventing Transfusion Errors

Each year, approximately 10 to 12 million red blood cell units are administered to individuals in the United States. Experts estimate that 0.1% of these transfusions result in a serious adverse event. Adverse events are estimated to lead to a short-term mortality of 1 to 1.2 per 100,000 individuals, or approximately 35 transfusion-related deaths per year. The long-term mortality, which includes disease transmission-related deaths such as AIDS, is estimated to be one per every 130,000 red blood cell transfusions, or approximately 85 transfusion-related deaths each year.[1,2] Although there certainly are instances of physicians administering blood, such as the surgeon in the operating room, the overwhelming majority of transfusions are administered and monitored by nursing staff.

Some transfusion errors do not result in adverse consequences. For example, due to clerical or communication errors, an individual receives a homologous transfusion before he or she receives a transfusion using available autologous (his or her own) blood units. While this error did not result in harm to the patient, it did go against the patient's wishes, and the organization's policy on using autologous blood units first was breached. Other transfusion errors are much more threatening. Transmission of HIV or hepatitis via blood transfusion, one type of transfusion sentinel event, has increased the public's perception of the risk of infection and intensified concerns about safety of the blood supply.

Another type of serious transfusion sentinel event is a hemolytic transfusion reaction (HTR). An HTR results in the destruction of an individual's red blood cells. The hemolysis or destruction is caused by an immunologic incompatibility between the donor and the recipient, or from non-immune mechanisms. Most HTRs result from the transfusion of ABO-incompatible red blood cells.[3] Reports put the incidence of fatal HTRs at 1 per 300,000 to 700,000 transfusions.[4] The incidence of ABO-incompatible transfusions is 1 per 33,000 units.[5] The immediate HTRs are usually due to clerical or systemic errors that result in the recipient receiving the wrong unit of blood. Factors that determine the severity of the reaction include the type of incompatibility, quantity of incompatible blood received, and period of time before initiating treatment for the reaction.

Data from the Joint Commission's Sentinel Event database indicates that transfusion errors accounted for 2.4% of all sentinel events reviewed by the organization between January 1995 and June 2001. A *Sentinel Event Alert* published in August 1999 reviewed data related to twelve of these cases, all but one of which involved HTRs.[6] Ten of the 12 transfusion errors were fatal. Eleven of the transfusion errors occurred in a general hospital with eight occurring in high-risk areas (that is, emergency departments, intensive care units, and operating rooms). One case occurred in a long term care facility. Reviewers noted that all of the processes involved in blood transfusion contain factors commonly acknowledged to increase the risk of an adverse outcome. These appear in Sidebar 3-1, page 38.

Root Causes and Prevention Strategies

Organizations that experienced a sentinel event related to a transfusion error reviewed by the

SIDEBAR 3-1. FACTORS INCREASING THE RISK OF ADVERSE OUTCOMES

Error experts have identified numerous factors that contribute to the risk of adverse events. Blood transfusion processes include each of these factors:

- *Variable input.* Individuals have different blood types.

- *Complexity.* Cross-matching, administering, and monitoring effects of the blood involve complex and technical processes.

- *Inconsistency.* Transfusion procedures are not standardized across health care organizations.

- *Tight coupling.* Blood transfusion requires multiple steps that occur so closely together that there is little opportunity for intervention if failure is noted. Interrupting process sequence, especially in an emergency department, operating room, or intensive care unit, is difficult if not impossible.

- *Human intervention.* Transfusion processes require a level of consistency not necessarily achievable by health care workers without computer support.

- *Tight time constraints.* Transfusions occur in high risk area, such as operating rooms, intensive care units, and emergency rooms, where speed is required.

Source: Joint Commission: Transfusion errors: Preventing future occurrences. *Sentinel Event Alert* Issue 10, Aug 30, 1999.

Joint Commission identified the following root causes:[6]

- Information-related factors: Patient identification, specimen label, or blood label errors or incomplete communication among caregivers.

- Patient assessment and monitoring: Incomplete patient blood verification or not recognizing the signs and symptoms of a transfusion reaction.

- Staff-related factors: Insufficient orientation and training or inadequate staffing levels.

- Equipment or environment of care-related factors: Unsafe storage procedures, such as blood for multiple surgical patients stored in the same refrigerator.

- Care planning: No informed consent for a transfusion.

- Laboratory procedures: Multiple samples cross-matched at the same time or a cross-match started before the order is received.

Eleven of the cases reviewed by the Joint Commission involved multiple failures to follow established procedures. The most frequent procedural failure was the verification of the blood recipient's identity with the correct unit of blood. Three cases involved handling either the blood samples or the units for more than one individual in the same location at the same time. A look at root causes and prevention strategies within the nursing domain follows.

Root Cause 1: Faulty Patient and Unit Identification/Verification Process

Sentinel Event Example: Faulty Verification. *In the operating room, an anesthetist requests a unit of red blood cells for a patient who already has lost a unit of blood, is continuing to lose blood, and is experiencing a decrease in blood pressure with an increased heart rate. The circulating nurse obtains a unit of blood and, working with the anesthetist, commences the required process for confirming the correct patient and blood unit. The circulating nurse has to interrupt the process to attend to an urgent request by the surgeon. The anesthetist completes the review of the blood slips without the circulating nurse and starts the transfusion.*

A couple of minutes later, the circulating nurse reviews the slips and labels and discovers that the transfused blood is intended for another patient with the same last name and a very similar identification number. Unfortunately, the patient already has received most of the unit. He develops a life-threatening intraoperative coagulopathy that does not respond to aggressive therapy.

The root cause analysis conducted following this sentinel event reveals that the participants involved did not recognize the serious risks involved with patient-unit identification, the need for consistency in the identification process, and the "tight coupling" requirements of not interrupting the identification sequence. Thereafter, organization policy required completion of the patient-unit identification process. If this process is interrupted, the entire sequence has to be repeated with the same or new caregivers.

Failure to properly identify a patient is a major factor in blood transfusion sentinel events. A properly designed and implemented identification process enables staff to match the proper unit of blood with the correct patient. A complete, thorough, and correct patient-blood verification policy and process is critical to patient safety. The transfusion policy must address identification of the specimen, the patient, and unit of blood. The policy and procedures must be developed collaboratively because invariably, they affect and involve more than one department. The organization's administration and medical staff should approve all collaboratively developed policies and procedures.

High quality and accurate patient-identification band procedures are key to solving the problem of matching the correct patient with the correct unit of blood. Some facilities use unique identification bands for patients receiving transfusions. The unique band must match the specimen tube and the labeled unit. Some kits provide a band, specimen label, unit label, chart label, order label, and transfusion record label all keyed to the same number. One system uses a wristband with a length of the band that extends beyond the section around the patient's wrist. The extended portion, which contains the patient's unique number, can be placed in a hand-held device from which a label can be printed. Organizations may also wish to consider bar coding systems which can help to reduce patient-blood verification errors.

Most verification processes are still too dependent on the observer visually checking both the patient's band and the unit's label. Ideally, in the future, an electronic device could be developed that would be used to confirm the verification. Computerized verification could not only identify the patient and unit of blood, but might also consider pretransfusion laboratory criteria.

Nurses play a key role throughout the transfusion process. They must be knowledgeable about verification policies and procedures and follow them consistently at all times. If nurses find that current policies and procedures are inadequate, they should alert appropriate parties and participate on teams charged with making improvements.

Prevention Strategies

Know the organization's procedure for identifying the patient. The patient identification process starts with securing the required identification information. This may not be as simple as it sounds, depending upon where and how the individual arrives in the organization. Perhaps the person arrives through the emergency department, by ambulance to a nursing facility, or through a transfer from a long term care facility. The confused or severely injured patient might not be identifiable on initial contact. What if the patient entered the system through the blood bank to provide autologous blood prior to the day of surgery? Or perhaps the individual is receiving the blood in an outpatient clinic. By being knowledgeable about how identification is initiated, the nurse can be better prepared to understand what is or is not acceptable. Ideally, the identification process should be consistent throughout the facility, or the process might be prone to errors. Nurses can help to identify process problems.

Know how identification information is documented organizationwide. The nurse should be aware of the specific data and information used to identify the patient in the clinical record and on a wristband, as appropriate. For example, the facility might require a name, birth date, room number, or social security number. Perhaps the facility provides a unique identifier such as a medical record number or a specific numbered transfusion wristband. Is there a different patient registration number and chart number? Nurses should know how to identify a patient for a transfusion and whether the process is uniform throughout the facility. Is it the same for inpatients and outpatients? The nurse should be aware of these additional identification possibilities, but recognize what must be used when transfusing blood according to the established policy.

Help to ensure proper specimen and unit labeling. Labeling is an essential process required in order to identify the specimen, and to enable the specific unit of blood to be transfused to the correct patient. Nurses and laboratory staff must precisely and properly execute each and every step in the labeling process. A complicated process that is used infrequently by the staff can result in errors. Staff in one organization used a separate blood transfusion wristband to identify the patient when a specimen was drawn. However, instead of having all the needed equipment (that is, wristband sleeve, wristband label, specimen container, labels, and needles) in one place or prepackaged, the nurses had to locate all the components. Although the separate banding was a good idea, the cumbersome process of trying to find all the appropriate components needed to make the identification process work was fraught with potential errors. In spite of frequent training sessions, the labeling error rate did not improve until staff redesigned the patient and blood unit identification process. They decided to use a prepackaged system that included all the components that the nurses would need.

Clarify any confusing patient identification procedures. One organization's patient identification verification transfusion policy stated that the nurse should write the patient's wristband identification number on the blood specimen label. The wristband had both a medical record number unique to the patient, and an encounter number unique for that admission. The staff was confused about which number to use as the "official" identification number. After the policy was clarified, some of the specimen tubes were still occasionally mislabeled. The facility changed to an addressograph label that was wrapped around the tube. However, now there was the risk of using the wrong addressograph label on the specimen.

Because the organization recognized the risk involved with the addressograph label, the

organization stressed in their education sessions the importance of replacing the addressograph cards in the proper slots, and double checking the labels before and after being applied. The staff was well informed that the addressograph label could be the weak link in the process, and about the need for vigilance when using the addressograph labels. The organization was considering a change to a separate blood transfusion banding system that would have prenumbered bands, labels, and forms.

Nurses should clarify any confusing patient identification procedures, alert organization leaders to these problems, and participate in redesigning procedures, as necessary.

Confirm the patient's name with the patient, and check the unique patient identifier on the wristband before administering blood. When the blood is available, the nurse must follow the established processes for obtaining and administering the unit of blood. This includes identifying the correct patient with the correct unit of blood. The unit of blood must be properly labeled to prevent the mismatch of recipient and donor blood. The nurse should check the label for the patient's name, unique identifier (hospital number, blood wristband number, etc.), the blood unit's unique identification number, ABO and RH type, and the expiration date. Prior to administering the unit of blood, the administering nurse and other caregivers involved in the blood's transfer from the lab should read aloud the information identifying the patient and the unit of blood. This confirmation is a mandatory part of the transfusion process. Confirmation should be documented by both individuals. Required information such as time and date and appropriate signatures must be provided.

In outpatient areas, health care providers must be careful in identifying patients in waiting rooms. Using both the name and the patient's birth date or social security number helps to decrease the possibility that patients with similar names are mistaken.

Alert supervisors about the use of problematic patient identifiers. Data have shown that using the care recipient's room number as the patient identifier is problematic. Some facilities attempt to distinguish between multiple individuals in the same room with letters such as "A" or "B" or "door" and "window" designations. However, this problem is compounded when patients are reassigned to different rooms during their stay.

Root Cause 2: Insufficient Communication/Information Availability

Sentinel Event Example: Lack of Communication Among Staff. *A patient is transported from her room to the cardiology suite for urgent echocardiogram studies. Immediately prior to transfer, she receives a transfusion of red blood cells. The transfusion information is documented in the nursing notes, which are reviewed when the patient is in the procedure room. The transport orderly is not aware of the recent transfusion. As customary, the patient waits on the stretcher outside the cardiology procedure room until her scheduled time. While waiting in the hall, she begins to experience signs and symptoms of a transfusion reaction. Since the cardiology suite staff is not yet aware of the recent transfusion, they do not recognize the symptoms' etiology and the urgency of the situation. Once the situation is recognized, the patient is transferred to the intensive care unit where she is successfully treated for the reaction.*

Review of the event reveals that methods to communicate relevant information are not available when patients were transported for various studies. Organization leaders revise the procedures. Unit nurses are now required to report any "special issues" concerning their patients to the staff that will be caring for the patient. This communication can be by telephone, or the nurse can accompany the patient to the site. The policy specifically lists the completion of a recent transfusion as a special issue that must be communicated. In addition, the orderlies transporting patients should also receive a report from the patient's nurse. Orderlies are required to immediately present the patients and the charts to the staff performing the studies. A newly developed transport document conveys critical information about recent transfusions, medications, signs, and symptoms.

Sentinel Event Example: Lack of Key Information. *In one facility using a clinical guideline protocol, patients provide autologous blood prior to specific elective procedures. At times, however, clinical indications with the patient prevent the phlebotomist from drawing the required units. In one instance, the phlebotomist cancels a blood draw because a patient's blood pressure is elevated. The patient subsequently receives treatment for his hypertension from his internist. His day of surgery arrives and he has provided only one of the two requested autologous units. The surgeon is not aware of this situation. The surgery is performed as scheduled. The patient requires a second unit of blood postoperatively. When the patient is later diagnosed with complications from hepatitis C virus (HCV), the source of the infection is determined to be the non-autologous unit of red blood cells.*

A review of the event reveals that the organization had established no routine mechanism for communicating to surgeons prior to the day of surgery whether the requested autologous units of blood were available for elective cases. If the surgeon had this information prior to the day of surgery, he and the patient could have decided whether this elective case should be rescheduled in order to give the patient additional time to provide the second autologous unit. Since the patient was concerned about the risks of transfusion-related infectious disease transmission, even if infrequent, the opportunity to reevaluate the situation should have been available to the patient.

Organizations experiencing transfusion sentinel events frequently cite incomplete communication among staff members and the failure to correctly transfer information as root causes. The availability of accurate information regarding the care recipient, blood units or specimens, and laboratory tests and timely and accurate communication of that information are critical to patient safety.

Informed consent is an important part of the information acquisition and communication process. How does the nursing staff at each organization participate in the informed consent process required for transfusions? Is the physician required to write a progress note explaining the situation, or does the patient sign a specific preprinted transfusion consent form? What are the state and/or medical staff regulations regarding informed consent? If the organization includes language for transfusion informed consent in the surgical consent, is it valid for the entire hospitalization and throughout the organization? How does a staff member document a patient's refusal to accept a transfusion? How is this information communicated to the rest of the staff? Nurses should know how to identify a patient with religious or cultural concerns about transfusions. How does the organization address religious concerns involving pediatric patients? These and other questions should be addressed in the organization's policies and procedures and through nurse training.

Frequently, patients want considerable information on the incidence of transfusion reactions, and the risk of getting AIDS, hepatitis, or other transfusion-related diseases. Organization leaders should ensure a mechanism by which the nurse can provide the patient with accurate information. Some organizations print detailed information on the back of transfusion-informed consent forms.

Prevention Strategies

Know how to access vital information. The transfusion process requires the availability of information concerning the patient's identification in the record, on orders, in the computer, on the specimen, on the unit of blood, and on the wrist or other band attached to the patient's body. Access to the patient's prior transfusion history is often very valuable. The nurse must know how to access all this information. If the information is not available, or the process is too cumbersome, the nursing staff should participate in collaborative efforts to improve the situation.

Ensure proper documentation and its use as a communication tool. One organization uses a transfusion documentation form that details the steps required prior to giving a patient a unit of blood. The sheet identifies the requirement for a consent form, solutions that can be used with the blood, specific filters that can or should be used for the various blood components, identification steps that require confirmation with another trained staff member, instructions given to the patient about possible symptoms, and the initial set of vital signs that are required. The nurse documents each step in boxes or sections. The instructions and training stress that each step should be documented when it is actually completed. Completing the form *after* the task is completed could allow one of the safeguards to be bypassed. Additionally, the form lists the signs and symptoms that require stopping the transfu-

sion and calling the physician. If the patient's physician determines that a transfusion reaction has occurred, then the steps for treating the reaction and initiating the investigation of the reaction can be found on the reverse side of the form. The forms are audited periodically to determine compliance, and opportunities to improve the process. Although documentation does not guarantee the steps are completed as intended, the absence of the documentation might identify a process problem.

Root Cause 3: Inadequate Patient Assessment and Monitoring

"Near Miss" Example: Inadequate Post-Transfusion Monitoring. *A patient is taken to the radiology department after a transfusion is started. The organization's transfusion policy does not address the monitoring requirements for patients when they are removed from their rooms during a transfusion. The patient develops urticaria and an increased temperature while in the radiology waiting area. Fortunately, the patient is able to ask for assistance and is transferred back to his room. The organization reviews its policy and makes provisions that would help to ensure that patients receiving blood are satisfactorily monitored regardless of location.*

Initial patient assessment ensures that a patient should actually receive blood. After the blood is administered, ongoing monitoring ensures that any adverse events are identified and treated promptly and appropriately. Nurses play a key role in confirming a thorough patient assessment that identifies the need for the transfusion. They also can identify a transfusion reaction, provide required treatment, and record and document monitoring results as outlined in organization policy.

Prevention Strategies

Confirm the need for the transfusion. Organizations often establish "transfusion criteria," used to determine whether a patient should receive blood. Staff audit the transfusion record to determine whether it is appropriate to give the patient a transfusion based on pre-determined laboratory values, and the clinical history. In some instances, a physician might want a patient who does not meet the laboratory criteria to receive blood if the physician feels there is a clinical indication. An astute nurse will check the laboratory values to see if the order for the blood meets the established criteria. If the hemoglobin, hematocrit, or platelet count is above the established criteria, the nurse can check the physician's notes to learn of the rationale for giving the transfusion. If there is still a question, a discussion with the physician could possibly save the patient from the risk involved in an unneeded transfusion. Some facilities are using an order sheet for blood transfusions that includes the transfusion criteria. If the values do not correlate, the physician can write an explanation of the reasons for the transfusion in the appropriate sections. In this scenario, if the nurse receives a verbal order from the physician for a transfusion, the nurse would be expected to complete the transfusion order form with the required information obtained from the physician.

Ensure the availability and communication of key assessment findings. Nurses are in an excellent position to help determine what information is required from the physician's assessment in order to safely provide the transfusion. Nurses in an outpatient transfusion unit must receive the information they need from the ordering practitioner. Other than the order, what additional information is provided? Nurses must be made aware of the patient with a history of congestive heart failure and how the fluid load will be handled with this patient. Nurses can advise about the information required to perform transfusions safely and efficiently. A collaborative effort with all departments involved will contribute to a successful system.

Monitor and observe the patient during and following a transfusion. Nurses must appropriately monitor a patient receiving a transfusion and promptly identify any transfusion reactions that occur. Failure to do so can result in treatment delay and, in the worst case, a sentinel event. Nursing staff must be able to recognize the signs and symptoms of a transfusion reaction. If appropriate training is not provided, nurses must request it and assure that they are properly trained prior to administering any blood. Training should address what to monitor, monitoring frequency and timing, and documenta-

tion. Some organizations provide a monitoring documentation form with the same identification information as on the unit's label. The staff then records monitoring data on the transfusion record, keeping the original for the chart, and returning a copy to the blood bank laboratory. Ancillary staff can also be trained to report visible patient symptoms and complaints to nurses so they can follow up on possible transfusion reactions more quickly.

Root Cause 4: Inadequate Staffing Levels, Orientation, Training, or Competence Assessment

"Near Miss" Example: Inadequate Staffing Level.
During the dinner period, only two nurses are available in one hospital wing. In order to expedite the transfusions needed for two patients, the nurses meet at the nursing station, review and confirm the patient-unit identification slips, and proceed to the patient's respective rooms to start the transfusions. While placing a unit of blood on the intravenous pole, one nurse notes from the unit's label that he has picked up the wrong unit. He runs quickly to the other patient's room and stops his colleague from administering the incorrect unit.

A review of this near miss event indicates that because of limited staff availability, the nurses bypassed normal procedures for verifying the proper patient and blood unit. The nursing policy stated that units should be checked at the bedside, not at a nursing station or outside the room. In addition, they were never to check more than one unit at a time. Their alternative actions had compromised the process requiring that identification and confirmation be conducted at the patient's bedside, and that two units were never to be checked simultaneously. The staff was instructed to contact the nursing supervisor on duty whenever staff availability prevented a procedure from being conducted according to organization policy.

Ensuring the appropriate number and level of nursing staff, trained and competent in transfusion policies and procedures, is critical to patient safety. Staff orientation, training, and competence assessment help to ensure an accurate patient/blood identification process, patient monitoring, identification of problems, and the ability to address problems. Leaders are responsible for ensuring appropriate and effec-

---

SIDEBAR 3-2. SAMPLE TRANSFUSION TRAINING TOPICS

- Autologous transfusions
- Transfusion criteria
- Advantages and disadvantages of component therapy
- Emergency transfusion prior to availability of cross-matched blood
- Use of platelets and plasma

- Use of cryoprecipitate or plasma derivatives
- Massive transfusions problems
- Equipment
- Use of volume expanders other than blood products
- Early recognition of transfusion reactions

---

tive staff supervision. Proper staff supervision involves developing, maintaining, and assessing staff competence and developing, implementing, and improving effective policies and procedures. In many organizations, nurses with extensive transfusion experience are responsible for training and supervising less experienced nurses.

Some transfusion error experts have suggested a staffing model that assigns a dedicated team to manage the transfusion procedure. This concept is similar to the use of teams for hyperalimentation, resuscitation, and conscious sedation. Although a dedicated team may not be possible, particularly in small organizations, leaders of all organizations need to identify nurses who require training and competence with transfusion procedures. Once these individuals are identified, leaders must provide them with the needed orientation, training, and ongoing competence evaluation. Basic training should cover the organization's transfusion policies and procedures, the use of equipment, and documentation requirements. Additional training topics that could be addressed appear in Sidebar 3-2, above.

Competence assessment is essential for a safe transfusion program. Written tests can only play a *part* in determining someone's knowledge base and judgment. Competence must also be assessed through *observation* of skills during actual transfusions. Observation and evaluation are useful processes for even the most experienced individuals. The observer might notice a

flawed practice that is not obvious to the individual performing the task.

Prevention Strategies

Follow established procedures throughout the transfusion process. The nurse's role in the transfusion process starts when he or she receives the order for blood. If a specimen previously has been collected, the nurse sends the request to obtain blood to the laboratory. If the laboratory requires a specimen to "type and cross" the blood, the nurse must be aware of her role in the process. In some organizations, all specimens are drawn by laboratory personnel. In this case, the laboratory is contacted and someone arrives to draw the blood. However, in other care settings, such as the emergency department or a skilled nursing facility, the nursing staff might be responsible for obtaining the specimen. The steps for identifying the patient, labeling the specimen, and sending the specimen to the laboratory for processing must be accomplished according to organization policy and procedures.

Learn about and understand the types of units being administered. Nurses should be familiar with blood unit types including autologous, homologous, and directed donor units. This knowledge provides an additional safeguard during the transfusion process. If a homologous unit is ordered, nurses can take an extra step to inquire about whether any lower-risk autologous units are available. Nurses should understand the policies concerning autologous transfusions and that such transfusions are not without risk, such as labeling or clerical errors. Often the autologous donation program is part of a clinical pathway.

Know and be competent in appropriate techniques for withdrawing blood from different types of invasive lines. Acquire and maintain high-quality phlebotomy skills. When withdrawing blood specimens from invasive lines, the nurse must be aware of proper sterile techniques, the aliquot of blood that must be removed before the specimen is obtained, and the proper techniques for flushing the lines. The nurse must know about the requirements for an intravenous catheter of the appropriate size and the correct electrolyte solution to be infusing when blood is administered. Leaders must provide an appropriate orientation and training program and a means by which to evaluate competence.

Root Cause 5: Unsafe Equipment or Environment of Care

Sentinel Event Example: Unsafe Blood Storage Procedures. *Following major abdominal surgery, a patient in a postanesthesia care unit (PACU) becomes hypotensive. His postoperative hemoglobin was reported to be quite low. While waiting to return to the operating room, the surgeon orders an immediate transfusion in the PACU using the blood remaining in the operating room refrigerator from the patient's earlier surgery. A unit clerk brings two units of blood to the PACU. Staff administer these to the patient without following the patient identification/blood unit matching procedures. One of the units of transfused blood stored in the operating room refrigerator was intended for another patient. The patient develops a hemolytic transfusion reaction and dies in the PACU.*

This example illustrates two failures: the failure to follow the organization's patient and unit identification/verification process and, critical to this section, the failure to follow established blood storage policies. All organizations should have a policy that addresses the storage of blood in refrigerators outside the laboratory. Although some facilities indicate that a refrigerator can only be used for one patient at a time, there is always the risk that someone will place additional units in the refrigerator, or that units might be left over from an earlier patient. Some policies indicate that if the unit of blood

requested is not used immediately, then the unit must be returned to the laboratory. Periodically, laboratories should survey sites to determine if refrigerators are available for the storage of blood. During one survey, a Joint Commission surveyor identified a refrigerator used for the storage of blood in a postanesthesia care unit (PACU) that was unknown to the pathology department. PACU nurses were not aware of the policy prohibiting the storage of blood in the refrigerator.

The organization described in the example above developed a new blood storage policy which prohibited refrigerators in operating room suites. Blood could be transported to the operating room only in patient-specific individual coolers. In addition, everyone in the operating room suite, including the unit clerk, received training on how to handle blood. A refrigerator in the operating suite, patient unit, or clinic, used to store multiple units for multiple patients, represents an error waiting to happen. This situation is particularly fraught with peril in high-risk areas, such as operating rooms or intensive care units where blood might be urgently sought and staff members hurried in their performance of key steps in the patient and blood unit identification/verification process.

Prevention Strategies

Know the organization's blood storage and handling policies and procedures. Nurses should follow these at all times.

Know how to use appropriate and available transfusion-related equipment. Equipment includes fluid warmers, filters, and infusion pumps. Any equipment can be misused or malfunction. Nurses must be oriented, trained, and competent in equipment use. Since many pieces of equipment have electrical components, nursing staff should be knowledgeable about alarm systems, preventive maintenance schedules, and electrical safety precautions.

Prevent contamination of blood products and equipment. Nursing staff also must act to prevent contamination of blood products and transfusion equipment during storage and handling. This requires training in how to handle and care for equipment. In addition, nurses should know how to recognize breeches in procedures that could contribute to contamination of the blood products or equipment.

Concluding Comments

Nurses can help prevent sentinel events due to transfusion errors. Proper education and training, a safe environment of care, adequate staffing and competence assessment, complete and timely patient assessment and monitoring, thorough communication, and a high quality patient/blood unit identification and verification process can increase the likelihood of safe transfusions.

References

1. Despotis G: Current and evolving issues in transfusion therapy. Park Ridge, IL: American Society of Anesthesiologists 1999 Annual Refresher Course Lectures, No. 162.

2. Goodnough LT, et al: Transfusion medicine: Blood transfusion. *New England Journal of Medicine* 340:438–447, 1999.

3. American Society of Anesthesiologists (ASA): *Questions and answers about transfusion practices,* 3rd edition. Park Ridge, IL: ASA, 1997.

4. Linden JV, et al: Decrease in frequency of transfusion fatalities. *Transfusion* 37:243–244, 1997.

5. Linden JV, Kaplan HS: Transfusion errors: Causes and effects. *Transfusion Medicine Reviews* 8:169–183, 1994.

6. Joint Commission: Transfusion errors: Preventing future occurrences. *Sentinel Event Alert* Issue 10, Aug 30, 1999.

Chapter 4:

Preventing Falls

According to the National Safety Council (NSC), nearly 3 million falls occur annually in homes, work, and all other settings in the United States. More than 16,600 of these were fatal, according to NSC data.[1] Fractures of the neck, femur, humerus, vertebrae, and other bones are common, as are soft tissue injuries such as hematomas, sprains, lacerations, and others. A "fall event" occurs when a person comes to rest inadvertently on the ground or other lower level, not as a consequence of sustaining a violent blow, loss of consciousness, or sudden onset of paralysis such as with a stroke or epileptic seizure.[2]

Cause for Concern

Falls resulting in injury are a fatal symptom. Beyond the fatality data cited above, the literature shows that the six-month mortality rate for octogenarians with a fall-created hip fracture, for example, is extremely high. Complications of hip fractures and bed rest during the recovery period include deep vein thrombosis, pulmonary embolism, and pneumonia. These are the killer syndromes. In addition, another severe consequence of falls is the individual's real and terrifying subsequent "fall-a-phobia." Fear can confine individuals who have fallen to an existence where they barely move. Muscles deteriorate, depression begins, eating slows, and there's a kind of slow death as quality of life further declines.

Falls are a serious problem in all health care organizations. They account for a significant proportion of injuries to hospitalized and ambulatory patients, long term residents, and home care and behavioral health care recipients. Falls frequently result in death and increased length and cost of hospital stays. In addition, they cause significant pain and suffering for individuals and their families and often lead to lawsuits.[3] Their costs are enormous. In-hospital falls were correlated with a 61% increase in total charges and a 71% increase in length of stay, not including costs of lawsuits or pain and suffering for the individuals involved.[3]

Fatal falls rank high on the list of sentinel events tracked by the Joint Commission.[4] Data from the Joint Commission Sentinel Event database indicate that falls accounted for 4.6% of sentinel events reviewed by the organization between January 1995 and January 2001. These occurred in 24-hour care settings; half of the falls involved individuals over the age of 80. Thirty-three percent fell from a bed; others fell while walking, in the bathroom, from a bedside commode, gurney, or chair. Another 33% of falls involved "extraordinary situations" like falling down a staircase, laundry chute, or from an upper story window, a roof, or a balcony.

A significant proportion of individuals who fell had an altered mental status due to acute or chronic illness (mental or physical), or acute intoxication. A history of prior falls, use of sedation, use of anticoagulant therapy, a recent change of environment, and urinary urgency were frequently associated risk factors either for the fall itself or for serious injury from the fall. Most of the falls occurred at night, weekends, and holidays—traditionally times of lower staffing levels.

Root Causes and Prevention Strategies

Organizations reporting fatal falls identified the following root causes:[4]

- Inadequate caregiver communication;
- Incomplete assessment or reassessment;
- Incomplete care planning and unavailable or delayed care provision;
- Staffing issues such as incomplete orientation and training of new staff, inadequate supervision of caregivers in training, and inadequate staffing levels;
- Environmental issues, such as unsafe window design, door locks, or nursing stations, or malfunction or misuse of equipment; and
- Insufficient education of care recipients and their families.

More than half of the organizations identified communication issues among caregivers as a root cause. These included failure to communicate information during nursing report, shift changes, or a transfer from a hospital to a nursing home; lack of documentation of changes in the individual's conditions in the clinical record; and inadequate communication from families regarding conditions and fall history. Forty-one percent of the organizations identified incomplete assessment and reassessment, incomplete care planning or lack of protocol, and environment of care issues as root causes.

Nurses play a critical role in the prevention of falls in all types of health care organizations. A close look at key root causes and prevention strategies follows.

Root Cause 1: Inadequate Caregiver Communication

Sentinel Event Example: Inadequate Staff Communication. *Two days following a surgical procedure, a hospitalized man begins to experience increased weakness, unsteady balance, and forgetfulness. Nursing staff on the 3:00 PM to 11:00 PM shift reassess the man and revise the plan of care. They do not verbally communicate this information to staff on the next shift; the assigned nurse leaves before changing the documentation on the plan of care. Since the 11:00 PM to 7:00 AM shift does not have the benefit of this information, a nurse helps the man into a chair for breakfast and leaves him unattended. When the breakfast tray is brought into the room an hour later, the man is found sitting on the bathroom floor bleeding from a large head wound.*

Communication and transfer of information between and among health care professionals are essential to reducing fall risk. In the previous example the incident could have been avoided if the man hadn't been left unattended for such a long time. Poor communication hindered the information flow from the evening to the night shift.

Coordinated communication can help staff to revise care plans appropriately and implement proactive fall risk reduction strategies. Thorough communication among nursing staff and other team members helps to ensure that care is provided in a coordinated manner. By observing the individual on a regular basis, nurses can identify changes in condition or behavior indicating problems or the need for care plan revision. Communication during shift changes or setting transfers is particularly critical. For example, a nurse on the day shift in a long term care setting must be informed by the night nurse that an individual receiving pain medication complained of dizziness. Ideally, communication should be both written and verbal. Thorough documentation in the clinical record of the care recipient's response to care and services must be ensured by nursing staff.

Prevention Strategies

Communicate, communicate, communicate. As mentioned in earlier chapters, nurses must communicate to all caregivers information concerning changes experienced by the care recipient. This must occur among all levels and all disciplines of staff, including administrative and environment of care staff.

Document, document, document. Documentation in the clinical record is essential and should be enhanced by a verbal report, whenever possible. Nurses can record on tape change-of-shift reports for the next shift staff. Use of a summary 24-hour report sheet that lists significant changes in condition as well as admissions and discharges is a helpful communication tool. This can be checked by the shift supervisor when making unit rounds and delivered to the nursing supervisor's office at the end of each 24-hour period. Nurses must ensure changes to the plan of care as soon as the needs and approaches have been established. Individuals at risk of falling can be identified in care plan documents by a color dot or other measure. To alert staff of fall risk, the dot can be placed over the head of the bed, on the chart, and at the entrance to the individual's room if regulations permit this. As always, be sensitive to the recipient of care's right to privacy and confidentiality of clinic information.

Root Cause 2: Inadequate Assessment and Reassessment

Sentinel Event Example: Inadequate Time For Assessment. *A man scheduled for a procedure requiring general anesthesia arrives at an ambulatory surgery center 30 minutes late for his preoperative assessment. The history and physical forwarded by his physician are brief. The nursing assessment is rushed and completed in a room full of distractions. As a result, neither the man nor his wife inform the nursing staff that certain anesthesia medications used during past operative procedures had changed his consciousness levels for a more prolonged period than normally expected.*

His surgery—the final one scheduled for the day—commences and proceeds without mishap. In the postoperative recovery area, the man exceeds the "usual" stay by one hour. Staff members again are rushed and anxious to complete their work for the day. Because the man responds verbally and is able to dress with minimal assistance from his wife, staff do not complete all steps in the postoperative assessment and discharge the man without identifying his residual mental confusion.

The man is wheeled out of the recovery area in a wheel chair and out the front door to where his wife is waiting. The wife leaves her husband sitting on a bench in front of the facility while she gets their car in an adjacent parking lot. After a minute or two, the man, not fully recovered from the effects of the anesthesia, becomes confused and attempts to walk alone to the parking area. He steps into oncoming traffic, is struck by a vehicle, and sustains a fractured hip.

Sentinel Event Example: Incomplete Assessment. *A 75-year old surgical patient with dementia is placed on a surgical unit following a routine procedure on his foot requiring general anesthesia. The nursing staff provides him with a wheelchair, and assumes that he is not at risk for injury since his*

room is close to the nursing station. This is within clear view and only ten feet from the elevator entrance. A member of the nursing staff is in the nursing station at all times.

At the end of the first morning on the unit, the man wheels himself to the far end of the unit where staff can no longer directly observe him. The man was found unconscious with multiple fractures after opening a closed fire door and falling down one flight of stairs in the wheelchair.

The first step in preventing falls is correctly and completely assessing and reassessing an individual's risk of falling. Many organizations build this risk assessment into the initial nursing assessment performed on admission. This assessment could include proper room or unit assignment for cognitively impaired individuals to areas where doors are locked or alarmed. Risk factors include history of previous falls, mental status, communication, sensory, and auditory deficits, medications, urinary alterations, and emotional upset. A full list of risk factors and medications that may predispose individuals to fall appears as Sidebar 4-1, page 50. The man in the example above was at risk for falls due to cognitive impairment and residual effects of anesthesia. In a study conducted by Donna J. Conley, RN, C, BSN, and colleagues in the mid 1990s, the risk factor "impaired judgment" in fact contributed the greatest relative risk of falling for hospitalized patients.[5]

A thorough reassessment process ensures that individualized interventions based on the initial assessment are meeting defined goals. Frequent monitoring lets team members know how the individual's status is changing. Observation of an individual's behavior is critical to reassessments conducted by nursing staff.

Prevention Strategies

Thoroughly assess and reassess the individual for fall risk. Health care leaders must ensure the assessment of each individual for fall risk as part of the interdisciplinary assessment process. Nurses assess for fall risk as part of the nursing assessment process. An initial assessment that fails to identify the individual's overall cognitive level, muscle strength, pain, and ability to perform activities of daily living can lead to invalid

SIDEBAR 4-1. RISK FACTORS FOR INJURIOUS FALLS AND MEDICATIONS THAT MAY PREDISPOSE INDIVIDUALS TO FALL

Risk Factors for Injurious Falls

- Previous falls
- Cognitive impairment
- Impaired balance, gait, strength
- Neurologic disease (for example, stroke, Parkinson's disease)
- Musculoskeletal disease (for example, arthritis, joint replacement, deformity, foot problems, sensory impairment)
- Chronic disease (for example, osteoporosis, cardiovascular disease, lung disease, diabetes)
- Impaired mobility
- Problems with nutrition
- Medications
- Number of prescription medications; greater than four associated with increased risk (for example, sedatives, antidepressants, neuroleptics, antihypertensive medications, diuretics)

- Addition of risk factors in someone already at risk (for example, introduction of new medications likely to affect balance, flare of chronic disease)

Medications that May Predispose Individuals to Fall

- Antiarrhythmics
- Antidepressants
- Antihypertensives
- Diuretics
- Hypoglycemics
- Laxatives
- Neuroleptics
- Nonsteriodal anti-inflammatory agents
- Psychotropics
- Sedatives/hypnotics
- Vasodilators

Source: Information excerpted from King MB, Tinetti ME: A multifactorial approach to reducing injurious falls. *Clin Geriatric Med* 12(4):745–759, Nov 1996. Used with permission.

conclusions about the individual's status. Assessing blood pressure while the individual is both sitting and standing for signs of insufficient blood flow and fainting is one effective proactive strategy. Thorough assessment enables nursing staff to suggest and implement a proactive approach to fall prevention as part of the care planning and provision processes.

Consider all medications as part of the assessment and reassessment processes. Nursing medication assessments and reassessments must take into account all prescription and over-the-counter drugs and supplements the individual is taking, medication allergies, and history of substance abuse, including abuse of tranquilizers or other prescription drugs. Nurses can advocate for physician and pharmacologist review of the use of benzodiazepines, especially those that are long acting, and limiting the use of these psy-

chotropic medications. Individuals with altered perception and cognition need aggressive and prompt assessment and regular reassessment from nursing staff. If an individual receiving behavioral health care services is not taking his or her medication as prescribed, his or her alertness level may change and he or she may experience the psychiatric symptoms the medication alleviated when taken properly. Too much or too little insulin will change an individual's blood sugar level and can lead to disturbances in thought, weakness, fainting, and dizziness. Some medications can cause dehydration in the elderly, which will also change mental status. These drugs are prescribed for various cardiac problems and can include blood pressure medication, cardiac drugs, and diuretics. Sedation used during outpatient surgery, in dental clinics, and some diagnostic testing can place individuals at risk for falls if they are not allowed to rest and are not receiving close observation from nursing personnel.

When indicated, use a combination of assessment techniques. Use of different assessment techniques, such as observation or communication with the individual and family, help to provide as thorough an assessment as possible. For example, Conley mentions that she assesses individuals for impaired judgment through both observation and communication techniques. "I ask individuals to get out of the wheelchair and walk to the bed so that I can observe the level of support they need to walk," describes Conley.[6] Later in the assessment process, Conley asks individuals whether they need help in walking. If they say "No," but she observes otherwise, she determines that they exhibit impaired judgment and are considered at increased risk of falling. This impaired judgment could be the result of an individual's cognitive impairment (from medication or another medical condition) or even from the individual's pride or sense of independence that prevents them from admitting that they need help.

Assess according to established criteria and use a risk assessment tool. Organization leaders must establish criteria, specific to their care recipient population, that place an individual at fall risk. Organizations frequently use an overall screening tool that includes fall risk along with other assessments such as nutrition and skin integrity. Assessment tools help raise awareness of the fall risk issue. Nurses may need to use these tools a second time if the patient becomes confused as the result of new medication or disruptions in daily routine. Nurses can help develop and implement tools specific to the population(s) served.

Obtain input from family members and educate care recipient and family about fall prevention strategies. Communication with family members and significant others is critical to thorough assessment of fall risk. Nurses should inform family members about factors that increase fall risk and inquire about the presence of any such factors. Educating the care recipient and family members about fall prevention strategies can help to reduce fall risk in the health care organization and after the individual is discharged. Techniques to improve strength and balance

are particularly critical. In some organizations, physical therapists will provide such education, which the nursing staff can reinforce.

Reassess regularly to ensure success of interventions and increased fall risk. Among other changes, medication changes, including drug additions and increased or decreased dosages, create the need for vigilant monitoring for possible new side effects. A new medication added to an individual's current medication regimen can cause dizziness, sedation, or some other symptom that places the individual at increased risk for falls. Regular nursing staff reassessment and monitoring for behaviors indicating impaired judgment, particularly if the individual has had any sort of procedure involving anesthesia, can reduce the risk of falls. Nurse monitoring of laboratory values for potential toxicity levels, which can cause changes in mental and physical ability, can also help prevent falls.

Increase awareness of processes related to dementia and appropriate care of individuals with dementia. In unfamiliar surroundings, individuals with dementia may experience an increased level of confusion at dusk and night. Called "sundowning," this is a high-risk time of day for falls for individuals with dementia. Nurses can develop care plans to address the assessed need to increase fall prevention measures at this time of day. Activities to redirect and divert the individual's attention can be provided, such as music, visitors, and pet therapy, as appropriate. Nurses can get additional information on caring for individuals with Alzheimers, one form of dementia, from the Alzheimer Association (*www.alz.org*).

Root Cause 3: Inadequate Care Planning and Provision

Sentinel Event Example: Incomplete Care Planning.
A man is admitted for behavioral health treatment. His physician's history and physical does not identify a previous allergy to Lithium. The man's guardian briefly states that, in the past, the man had been on numerous medications for his psychiatric condition and that he may have had reactions to some of the drugs. Since the information was vague at best, the nurse does not identify or document any allergies and completes the man's plan of care without addressing past medication sensitivity. The psychiatric resident

on call orders Lithium after reviewing the man's record. Within four hours, the man is found unconscious in the day area of the facility, having fallen and broken an arm and hip.

Sentinel Event Example: Inadequate Care Provision.

A home health nurse visits a 69-year-old woman recovering from hip replacement surgery. The nurse's role is to monitor the condition of the woman's hip incision, reinforce exercises ordered by a physical therapist, and help the woman learn to use a new walker recommended by the physical therapist for ambulation. During her first visit, the nurse assesses the woman and her needs. The nurse does not follow the care plan and assists the woman with ambulation, providing contact guard assistance rather than helping with the walker. The woman had used the walker prior to surgery, but during her hospitalization a neighbor had borrowed it. Unfortunately, the neighbor changed the walker's height and, having damaged one of the four wheels, replaced it with a smaller wheel. After the nurse leaves, the woman attempts to use the walker and falls, breaking her arm during the fall. Review of the nurse's narrative notes confirms the nurse's failure to redirect the woman to ambulate using the walker and to ensure that the walker is in working order and appropriately fitted.

The first example demonstrates the importance of a thorough medication assessment on admission of individuals receiving care. Undocumented medication allergies place an individual at increased risk of adverse drug reactions and increased risk of resulting falls. As demonstrated in the second example, the prevention of falls requires a multifactorial, interdisciplinary approach. After an individual has been identified as at-risk for falls, a multidisciplinary team should begin the care planning process and provide care according to the care plan. The nursing care plan is generally the first step in this process and is followed by additional disciplines, as determined by the care recipient's needs. Medical, nursing, pharmacy, and physical/occupational therapy staff participate in many care settings.

For example, interventions for an individual at risk of falling due to poor vision include balance and gait training by physical therapists, low vision aids from optometrists, and environmental safety assessment by nursing and occu-

pational therapy staff. Interventions for a person at risk of falling due to foot problems may include foot care by podiatrists or orthopedic staff, adaptive devices and proper shoes from occupational therapy and nursing staff. Interventions for an individual at risk of falling due to polypharmacy include selection of medications that are least associated with fall risk and prescription of the lowest effective dose with the shortest action by pharmacy and medical staff and monitoring by nursing staff.

The role of pharmacists and prescribers in team-oriented care planning is particularly critical due to the high correlation between falls and medication use. Pharmacists can identify specific drugs and drug categories that are associated with such fall risk factors as confusion, orthostatic hypotension, and dizziness. Pharmacists must alert interdisciplinary team members of the potential adverse risks associated with particular medications and work closely with physicians to determine whether continuation of the medication(s) in question is desirable given associated risks and treatment goals. They not only play a key role in educating nurses and physical and occupational therapists about symptoms to look for in individuals taking medications that increase the risk of falls, but also alert team members about specific monitoring parameters.

Prevention Strategies

Tailor fall prevention strategies to the individual's unique needs. Prevention strategies must be highly individualized. A care recipient's family members may be able to provide information on the individual habits and activities that could help to individualize these strategies. Some combined assessment and care planning tools enable nursing staff to select appropriate interventions based on the individual's risk level. In some cases, staff may need to adjust medications; in other cases, walkers or assistance or anything in between may be needed. For example, frequent toileting is an effective intervention for cognitively-impaired individuals and those on diuretics. "The former don't realize that they need help in getting to the toilet," notes Jane E. Mahoney, MD, assistant professor of medicine in the geriatric section of the University of

Wisconsin Medical School.[6] Falls on the way to the bathroom account for a large proportion of all falls in hospitals. Assisting with toileting when individuals receive diuretic medications, tranquilizers, or sedatives reduces fall risk. Also, giving diuretics to individuals while they are awake and active rather than before they go to sleep can prevent falls that occur when tired individuals must get out of bed to use the bathroom.

In numerous instances, falls result when an individual tries to get out of bed. In some long term care facilities, staff place mattresses on the floor so that residents have less distance to fall if they roll off the bed. Organizations also are beginning to purchase electric beds which allow the bed height to decrease to six to eight inches from the floor. For individuals with Huntington's disease, which causes random, spasmodic movements while individuals are sleeping and awake, adult size enclosed beds are used with success. One side rail can be left down, the bed placed in a low position and a large mat placed by the bed.

Help to ensure the provision of timely care. Timeliness of care has a significant impact on reducing fall risk. Many care recipients fall on the way to requesting nurse or other caregiver assistance. They may attempt to walk without required help when they are trying to alert the nursing staff to their need for toileting or pain control medication. By tracking the amount of time taken to answer call lights and decreasing response time, a number of organizations have noted a decreased number of falls linked to decreased response time.[7] Improved and standardized nurse call systems can reduce fall likelihood, as can administering pain medications before transfers or ambulation to decrease discomfort and allow for increased mobility and toileting according to a schedule established with the care recipient.

Recognize fall risk associated with restraint use and eliminate restraint use whenever possible. Studies conducted in the long term care community in the 1990s indicated that although the number of falls might have been higher initially in a restraint-free environment, injury severity declined significantly.[8, 9, 10] Restraint can increase the risk of harm and actually cause harm to indi-

viduals. Because muscles are not being used, prolonged use of restraints can decrease an individual's muscle strength and thereby increase the likelihood of falls and injury from falls when the individual is not in restraints. In addition, the use of restraints can increase fall risk as individuals try to escape their restraint. For example, an individual trying to get out of a bed with full bed rails might experience a more serious fall than if split bed rails were used. Between 1985 and 1999, 315 incidents of individuals getting caught, trapped, entangled, or strangled in beds with rails, resulting in death or injury, were reported to the FDA.[11]

The Hospital Bed Safety Workgroup, with representatives from more than 25 health care organizations, including the Joint Commission and companies providing products and services to health care organizations, encourages health care organizations to assess patients' needs and to provide safe care without restraints.[11] A half rail in the up position at the head of the bed will help prevent individuals from rolling out of bed, while a lowered half rail at the foot of the bed will let them get out of bed when needed. If individuals should not get out of bed without assistance, bed alarms can be used to alert staff to the individual's movement. Alternatives to bed rails suggested by the group appear in Sidebar 4-2, page 54. Effective alternatives to restraints exist in all health care settings. Nursing staff should be knowledgeable about alternative safe and appropriate interventions. If restraints are necessary, nursing staff should ensure that they are properly used.

Root Cause 4: Inadequate Staffing, Orientation, Training, and Supervision

"Near Miss" Example: Inadequate Staffing Level. *A large health care organization is experiencing the effects of flu season. The census is increasing as is the number of staff out ill. A geriatric unit needs one full time registered nurse in addition to a nurse manager. In an effort to make the budgeted bottom line more positive, the nurse manager does not request a replacement registered nurse when the nurse covering the 7:00 AM to 3:00 PM shift calls in ill. The nurse manager does offer to assist on the unit. However, she is called into meetings at 10:00 AM and is not able to return to the unit. During lunch, when all but one*

SIDEBAR 4-2. ALTERNATIVES TO USING BED RAILS

In most cases, care recipients can remain safely in bed without the use of bed rails. The following ideas can be implemented to avoid using bed rails:

■ Check on care recipients frequently. Often, close observation can prevent falls better than bed rails.

■ Use adjustable beds that can be raised and lowered to make it easier for care recipients to get in and out of beds and easier for staff to assist in this process.

■ Use transfer or mobility aids.

■ For individuals at a high risk for falls, put mats next to the bed to absorb impact when falls do occur. However, make sure that the mats do not increase the risk of falls due to tripping or uneven footing.

■ Identify reasons why individuals get out of bed including hunger, thirst, needing to use the bathroom, restlessness, insomnia, and pain. Try to meet these needs on a predictable schedule that care recipients are aware of and have input in to.

Source: Adapted from Hospital Bed Safety Workgroup: *A Guide to Bed Safety: Bed Rails in Hospitals, Nursing Homes, and Home Health Care: The Facts.* Web site: www.fda.gov/cdrh/beds/

---

nursing aide are taking a lunch break, three care recipients fall while attempting to get to the bathroom without assistance. All three individuals state that their request for assistance via the call lights had not been met for a long time, so they attempted to make the walk unassisted due to their urgent need to use the bathroom. Fortunately, none were severely injured.

Sentinel Event Example: Inadequate Orientation, Training, and Competence Assessment. *Due to staff illnesses, a nurse normally working in the emergency area is assigned to the day surgery unit. The nurse informs his supervisor that he has not worked in the day surgery area for more than two years and does not feel prepared or competent to do so. His supervisor states that it is his turn to go and reminds him that he passed a written test of cross department tasks last year and hence, is competent.*

Unfamiliar with discharge criteria and assessing day surgery patients, the nurse discharges a man too early. Without assistance, the individual is allowed to get up and begin dressing to return home. The moment the nurse leaves the room, the man's already low blood pressure drops even lower and he falls to the floor, breaking a leg. The nurse returns and finds the man on the floor breathing shallowly. He quickly calls for and receives assistance to move the man back onto a stretcher, and reassess and treats his condition.

Maintaining adequate staffing levels is a key area of concern in preventing falls. Organization leaders must provide sufficient staff to meet the needs of individuals served. Without adequate staffing, care recipients receive less assistance when needed, and care giving staff members receive less training and less supervision. These factors have a significant impact on the number and severity of falls. All care staff must be competent in addressing age-specific needs of care recipients and be trained to identify cognitive impairments, gait instability, or other conditions that place individuals at risk for falls. If an organization has a falls prevention program, all staff must be competent in program elements before providing care to individuals at risk of falling.

Prevention Strategies

Understand the physiology of falls. Nurses must be well versed in the physiology of falls. As described by Russell Massaro, MD, executive vice president for Joint Commission Accreditation Operations, "A fall is an assault on the normal physiology that keeps humans upright. Staying upright or walking are beautifully complex processes, integrating functions of the eyes, ears, sense of touch, neuromuscular system, nervous system, and cognitive abilities. These functions work together to create a dance in which walking is actually controlled falling. Every step a person takes is the beginning of a fall because gravity always wants us to fall."[6] Now consider a person who has abnormalities of the feet, like bunions or flat feet. Or perhaps the person wears bifocals or takes medications for hypertension, depression, or some other problem. This person is at increased risk of falling. "A fall is usually the result of the confluence of effects of multiple minor challenges to the delicate balance that keeps us upright," says Massaro.[6] Singular, simple answers do not assist assessment or prevention efforts. Nurses must understand the full realm of the fall prevention challenge.

Know fall risk factors. Nurses must be knowledgeable about fall risk factors. Studies that correlate specific disease states and other factors, such as medications with increased fall risk, abound in the health care literature. Nurses should be familiar with identified fall risk factors, such as the knowledge that adults taking more than three or four medications—polypharmacy—are at increased risk of recurrent falls. See Sidebar 4-1, page 50, referenced earlier in this chapter.

Know who is at risk for falling and implement the organization's fall prevention program. Thorough assessment and use of successful intervention techniques are critical in identifying those at risk of falling and implementing the organization's fall prevention program. Education of the family and significant others about safety strategy can help reduce the risk of falls in the facility and after the individual is discharged. Nurses must be well versed in effective education techniques. In addition, knowledge of how to effectively communicate fall risk, fall prevention strategies, and change in care recipients' conditions are critical to fall prevention.

Inform supervisor of unsafe staffing situations. As mentioned in previous chapters, as advocates for the individuals in their care, nurses should communicate their concern about unsafe staffing situations. Notification of a supervisor and documentation through channels established by the organization are appropriate.

Root Cause 5: Unsafe Environment of Care

Sentinel Event Example: Unsafe Environment for Patient Population. *An organization provides subacute care to individuals with AIDS, many of whom have AIDS-related dementia. Care is provided in a unit on the third floor of a multi-story building. Care recipients generally are ambulatory, except those in the final disease stage. Unit windows open ten inches.*

During early morning rounds, the nursing staff are not able to locate one individual. A nurse notes that one of the windows in the individual's room is open as far as it could be. Simultaneously, a visitor finds the man outside the facility, having fallen three floors while attempting to leave the building. He was so thin that he was able to work his way out the window and so confused that he did not realize that his room was on the third floor. Staff who installed the windows were not aware of how thin and emaciated AIDS patients could become. While the fall did not prove fatal, the individual had significant injuries requiring an extended acute care stay.

This example illustrates the importance of a safe environment of care. Organization leaders must ensure planning for a safe environment and implementation of a safety plan. Safety efforts should include making regular environmental rounds to check for possible hazards such as those that could contribute to falls. Individuals conducting these rounds should be trained to ensure safety compliance in all areas, including care units.

Participation of nurses on environmental rounds can help to reduce potential environmental hazards. For example, nurses are well equipped to identify problems that could lead high-risk care recipients to fall while trying to ambulate without assistance. Improved environmental assessment by nursing staff on the AIDS unit described above could have helped to prevent the man's fall while attempting to elope. Increased education of the environmental and safety staff of the conditions of individuals with AIDS might also have helped to prevent this fall.

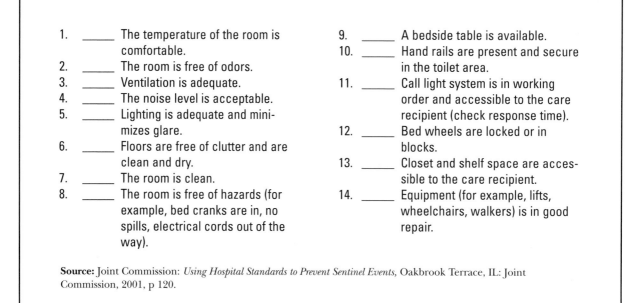

SIDEBAR 4-3. ENVIRONMENTAL CHECKLIST TO IDENTIFY FALL RISKS

1. _____ The temperature of the room is comfortable.
2. _____ The room is free of odors.
3. _____ Ventilation is adequate.
4. _____ The noise level is acceptable.
5. _____ Lighting is adequate and minimizes glare.
6. _____ Floors are free of clutter and are clean and dry.
7. _____ The room is clean.
8. _____ The room is free of hazards (for example, bed cranks are in, no spills, electrical cords out of the way).

9. _____ A bedside table is available.
10. _____ Hand rails are present and secure in the toilet area.
11. _____ Call light system is in working order and accessible to the care recipient (check response time).
12. _____ Bed wheels are locked or in blocks.
13. _____ Closet and shelf space are accessible to the care recipient.
14. _____ Equipment (for example, lifts, wheelchairs, walkers) is in good repair.

Source: Joint Commission: *Using Hospital Standards to Prevent Sentinel Events*, Oakbrook Terrace, IL: Joint Commission, 2001, p 120.

Prevention Strategies

Help ensure basic environmental safety. While housekeeping staff are ultimately responsible for keeping the care environment clean and tidy, nurses can play a key role in ensuring a safe environment of care. Areas used by care recipients must be clean and free of clutter. They also must be free of spills and loose cords or wires that could trip care recipients, staff, or visitors. Slippery floors lead to falls in all types of health care settings. A nurse aware of floor conditions, such as wetness caused by people bringing in moisture from outside, or a housekeeping person not mopping floors in correct manner so as to leave a dry path to walk on, can take actions to address the unsafe conditions. They also can advise care recipients and family members to take extra caution.

Equipment used by care recipients, such as wheelchairs, walkers, and canes, must be in proper repair (see prevention strategy, above). Properly fitting footwear allows for safe ambulating. A checklist developed by nursing staff and used when conducting weekly environmental rounds to identify and prioritize problems that could lead to falls appears as Sidebar 4-3, above.

Be knowledgeable about the organization's preventive maintenance program and vigilant about equipment needs and concerns. Nursing staff should know how to check equipment used by individuals receiving care for safety considerations and know how to notify maintenance of equipment needs and concerns. Organization leaders must ensure staff training about how to identify unsafe equipment, and the required steps to remove unsafe equipment from use.

Be particularly alert to unsafe bathrooms. As mentioned earlier, falls frequently occur in bathrooms or on the way to bathrooms in all types of health care settings. Older individuals who have not been able to go to the bathroom due to long waits for tests, crowded bathrooms, or delayed toileting assistance may not be able to control bladder functions well. The result may be dribbled urine while getting on or off the toilet. This represents a safety hazard. Non-skid floor coverings in toileting areas can help reduce fall risk and can be recommended by nursing staff. Nursing staff can be aware when individuals may need additional assistance with getting on and off the toilet. Some individuals are too embarrassed to request help, particularly if they are in an outpatient area like lab or x-ray, and can be asked whether they need assistance in a manner that ensures their privacy.

Use safety devices properly. When properly used, bed alarms, self-latching devices on utility rooms, exit alarms, "low beds" for those at risk for falls, locking bed wheels, and hand rails can significantly reduce the risk of falls in every organization. Some organizations use bracelets worn by individuals at risk of falling as an extra safety precaution to prevent individuals from leaving the appropriate area. The bracelet triggers a door alarm, alerting staff if the individual approaches and attempts to open the door.

Use fall prevention environment-of-care protocols established by the organization. Nurses should identify individuals at high risk of falling and provide additional environmental safety measures as outlined by organization leaders. Protocols might address such items as not allowing postsurgical patients to be up and about without supervision or staff assistance for a defined number of hours following surgery and encouraging family members to visit in "shifts" to help monitor the individual's status. When designing space, some organizations adopt a pod configuration in which the nursing station is located in the center of radiating rooms. Individuals at high risk of falling and others requiring maximum observation receive beds closer to the nursing station.

Concluding Comments

Fall-related sentinel events are a serious concern for all health care organizations. Nurses can help reduce the likelihood of deaths or serious injuries resulting from falls by improving caregiver communication, adequately assessing and reassessing individuals in their care for fall risk, thoroughly planning for and providing individualized care, ensuring competence in fall risk factors and prevention strategies, and helping to ensure a safe environment of care.

References

1. National Safety Council: Injury Facts-1998 Edition. Web site: *www.nsc.org/lrs/statinfo/99008.htm.*

2. Gibson MJ: The prevention of falls in later life. *Danish Medical Bulletin*, 34(4):1–24, 1987.

3. Bates DW, et al: Serious falls in hospitalized patients: Correlates and resource utilization. *Am J of Med* 99:137–143, Aug 1995.

4. Joint Commission: Fatal falls: Lessons for the future. *Sentinel Event Alert*, Issue 14, Jul 12, 2000.

5. Conley D, Schultz AA, Selvin R: The challenge of predicting patients at risk for falling: Development of the Conley Scale. *MEDSURG Nursing* 8(6): 348–354, Dec 1999.

6. Joint Commission: Catch them before they fall with multidisciplinary care plans. *Jt Comm Benchmark* 2(12):1–3, Dec 2000.

7. Joint Commission: *Using Hospital Standards to Prevent Sentinel Events,* Oakbrook Terrace, IL: Joint Commission, 2001, p. 114.

8. Strumpf NE, Evans LK: Alternatives to physical restraints. *J Ger Nurs* 18(11):4, 1992.

9. Evans LK, Strumpf NE, Williams C: Redefining a standard of care for frail older people: Alternatives to routine physical restraint. In Katz P, Kane R, Mezey R (eds): *Advances in Long Term Care.* New York: Springer, 1991, pp 81–108.

10. Evans LK, Strumpf NE: Myths about elder restraint. *Image: J of Nurs Scholarship* 22(2):124–128, Summer 1990.

11. Hospital Bed Safety Workgroup: *A Guide to Bed Safety: Bed Rails in Hospitals, Nursing Homes, and Home Health Care: The Facts.* Web site: *www.fda.gov/cdrh/beds.*

Chapter 5:

Preventing Infant Abductions and Release to Wrong Families

The issues of infant abduction and discharge to the wrong family have received increased attention by both the health care community and the general public due to well-publicized events in recent years. Infant abductions from hospitals are "emotionally devastating to new parents and the health care professionals who are charged to care for newborns," says John B. Rabun, Jr., ACSW, vice president and COO of the National Center for Missing & Exploited Children (NCMEC).[1] The organization's most recent data indicate that there were 104 infant abduction cases in health care facilities from 1983 to 1999.[2] More than half of the abductions from hospitals occurred from the mother's room and the rest from nursery, pediatrics, and on-premises settings. Ninety-eight of the infants were located, while six are still missing.

But there is some promising news. Between 1991 and 1998, there was a 55% reduction in infant abductions from health care facilities. In 1999, there were no reported abductions. "This reduction seems directly attributable to seven years of proactive-education programs combined with the use of electronic security measures," notes Rabun.[3]

Since the Joint Commission began tracking sentinel events in January 1995, the Accreditation Committee of the Joint Commission's Board of Commissioners has reviewed 20 cases related to infant abduction or discharge to the wrong family or the wrong family member. Most of the abductions took place in hospitals with more than 400 beds. The majority of the events occurred in the mother's room, followed by the newborn nursery and neonatal intensive care unit (NICU). Most of the infants were recovered unharmed within a few hours, and there was no evidence of violence to the mother or child. Most of the abductors were female. See Sidebar 5-1, page 60, for a profile of the "typical" abductor. In a number of cases, a woman impersonated a nurse or aide. In other cases, a woman pretended to be a volunteer, physician, or the infant's mother. In some cases, the birth mother abducted a child that was in the state's custody. Infants were abducted when taken for testing, during return to the nursery, when left unattended in the nursery, or while a mother was napping or showering. A number of the hospitals reported the discovery of failed abduction attempts shortly before the abduction occurred.

Despite these different circumstances, the root causes that have been identified provide insight into strategies nurses and other health care team members can use to reduce the risk in any infant abduction.

Root Causes and Prevention Strategies

Organizations that experienced an infant abduction reviewed by the Joint Commission identified the following root causes:[4]

- Physical environmental factors such as no line of sight to entry points as well as unmonitored elevator or stairwell access.
- Security equipment factors such as security equipment not being available, operational, or used as intended.
- Inadequate care recipient education.
- Staff-related factors such as insufficient orientation, training, competence assessment, or credentialing and insufficient staffing levels.

SIDEBAR 5-1. A PROFILE OF THE "TYPICAL ABDUCTOR"

1. Female of "childbearing" age (range 12–50 years); often overweight.
2. Most likely compulsive; often relies on manipulation, lying, and deception.
3. Frequently indicates that she has lost a baby or is incapable of having one.
4. Often married or cohabitating; companion's desire for a child may be the motivation for the abduction.
5. Usually lives in the community where the abduction takes place. Frequently initially visits nursery and maternity units at more than one healthcare facility prior to the abduction; asks detailed questions about procedures and the maternity floor layout; frequently uses a fire exit stairwell for her escape; and may also move to the home setting.
6. Usually plans the abduction, but does not necessarily target a specific infant; frequently seizes on any opportunity present.
7. Frequently impersonates a nurse or other allied healthcare professional.
8. Often becomes familiar with health care personnel and even with the victim parents.
9. Demonstrates a capability to provide "good" care to the baby once the abduction occurs.

Source: Developed by the National Center for Missing & Exploited Children from an analysis of 187 cases occurring 1983–1997. Used with permission.

- Communication and information-related factors such as delay in notifying security when an abduction was suspected, improper communication of relevant information among caregivers, improper communication between hospital units, and birth information published in local newspapers.

- Organization cultural factors such as reluctance to confront unidentified visitors or providers.

All of the organizations cited unmonitored entry or exit points or an unsafe environment of care as a root cause of the sentinel event. More than 60% of the organizations identified a lack of security equipment as a root cause. Approximately 50% cited staff orientation or training, care recipient education, and communication as root causes. Figure 5-1, above, provides a graphic look at the frequency of each type of root cause.

Discharge to the wrong family has occurred across the country in both urban and rural settings. The primary cause cited for this sentinel event has been improper identification of the infant and mother. This may be due to failure to follow identification procedures, equipment failure, or inadequate staff orientation and training. There also have been cases entailing the deliberate switching of infant identification bands by men who may be involved in paternity suits in order to avoid child support.

Organizations must develop and implement a proactive infant abduction and release to wrong family prevention plan. The nurses' role is essential in identifying not only potential abductors and means of escape, but also in correctly identifying the correct family or person that should be the recipient of the infant or child upon discharge. The nurse is with the mother, infant, and family more than any other staff member and often becomes aware of potential problems.

Leaders must support the active role of the nurse in the development of a proactive infant security program. Too often, infant abduction programs are developed and implemented without nurses' involvement. Nursing expertise and "buy in" are critical. Organizations have produced high quality, comprehensive, and proactive infant abduction policies and procedures by involving nurses from the obstetrical area, NICU, pediatrics, emergency department, and surgery. One such policy appears as Figure 5-2, page 64.

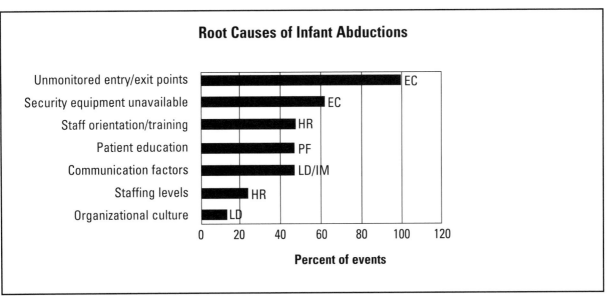

Figure 5-1. *This chart illustrates the percentage of causes at the root of infant abductions reported to the Joint Commission between January 1995 and January 2001.*

A closer look at each root cause cited earlier will help to identify strategies nurses can use to reduce the likelihood of infant abductions or release to wrong families.

Root Cause 1: Unsafe Environment of Care; Faulty or Unavailable Security Equipment

Sentinel Event Example: Unsafe Environment of Care. *A 45-year-old female enters the obstetrical unit of a community hospital on a Sunday evening. She knows the unit's routines because she has visited a number of times. She also is knowledgeable about the hospital's security systems, exits, and staff. She tours the unit, noting which rooms both mothers and newborns occupy. She also notes the presence or absence of visitors in each room. She identifies a private room occupied only by a young mother and newborn. She chats with a visitor in the hallway while keeping an eye on the room. As she is doing so, the new mother leaves her sleeping newborn unattended in a bassinet, steps into the bathroom and closes the door. The woman enters the room, puts the infant in a body carrier under her coat, and exits undetected through a back stairwell.*

The hospital uses security sensors on infant arm bands, but the detectors for the sensors are limited to the main egress corridor. The two remote exit doors are locked to prevent entrance from the outside but they are not secured to prevent egress. The unit is on the ground floor of the hospital and none of the windows are secured nor are they equipped with sensor detectors.

Health care organizations are required to plan for and provide a safe environment of care. Safety embraces planning and providing for a secure environment to protect care recipients, visitors, and staff. Access to the facility and unit must be controlled. The example described here indicates what can happen when an organization has not provided a safe care environment. Russell L. Colling, a health care security consultant in Salida, Colorado, recommends that hospitals use a designated public entry point and restrict access to all other entry points.[4] Large units can have a secondary entry point, but there should also be a closed-circuit television system with a videotape record at that entrance. Other experts advise organizations to have only one exit that is used for discharge of mothers and newborns. Security mechanisms or equipment must be available, operational, and used as intended. For example, security cameras must be positioned for high-quality visualization of the units and to better assess any unusual activity.

The Joint Commission suggests that hospitals consider the following actions in the environment of care and equipment arenas[4]:

■ Attach secure identically numbered bands to the baby (wrist and ankle bands), mother, and father or significant other immediately after birth.

Sample Infant and Child Abduction Policy

PURPOSE: To provide for the safety and security of all infants and children in the hospital. The hospital is also dedicated to having a proactive approach to reduce the risk of infant and child abduction. There is a systematic approach to increase awareness/prevention and to detect and manage an infant or child abduction. All areas of the organization are included in this policy with special emphasis on those areas providing services to infants and children.

PROCEDURE:
- All employees of the organization will receive education during orientation related to the organization's infant/child abduction prevention strategies including "Code Stork" and are trained as "Code Stork Assistants."
- There will be a minimum of three drills for "Code Stork," one per shift, each year.
- Infant and child abduction awareness and updates will be included in the annual mandatory in-services.
- Uniformed personnel with proper identification badges only may transport infants and children.
- If a parent transports the infant/child, an appropriate hospital employee must accompany them.
- The organization will not provide the local media/newspapers with birth notices.
- Security numbered bands will be attached to the baby (wrist and ankle bands), mother, and father or significant other immediately after birth.
- Footprints of the baby and a record of the baby's physical examination will be documented within the first hour of birth.
- Staff are required to wear up-to-date, conspicuous, color photograph identification badges.
- Access to the to nursery/postpartum unit will be by swipe-card locks and video surveillance will be at all access points including the emergency department, pediatrics, ICU, and nursery/postpartum.
- An infant security sensor system will be used for all infants and children under the age of five.

CODE STORK PROCEDURE
1. Notify the hospital operator—#999—and give the location of the abduction and description of the infant/child.
2. The hospital operator will call "Code Stork" and briefly describe the infant/child.
3. The operator will notify the appropriate leaders: CEO, V.P. Patient Care Services, Risk Manager, Physician, and Security Officer.
4. All entrances and means of egress will be secured and or manned. All bags, packages and means of concealment will be searched.
5. All staff will act as "assistants" and will look for anyone carrying, concealing or traveling with an infant/child. Staff will attempt to stop the person from further movement unless this might put them in danger. In this case they will be responsible for getting an accurate detailed description of the person. They will keep a safe distance and note the means of escape. If the abductor uses a car, the make and model, color, and license of the car needs to be noted, if possible.
6. Notify the operator of your findings and the operator will immediately notify security.
7. Continue to search and if anything is found, protect the scene to preserve evidence. Notify security immediately.
8. The hospital operator will call an "all clear" when the "Code Stork" incident is ended.

Figure 5-2. *Sample infant and child abduction policy.* **Source:** *Used with permission of Joan Dodelin.*

- Footprint the baby, take color photographs of the baby, and record the baby's physical examination within two hours of birth.

- Require staff to wear up-to-date, conspicuous, color photograph identification badges.

- Consider options for controlling access to nursery/postpartum unit such as swipe-card locks, keypad locks, entry point alarms or video surveillance. Any locking systems must comply with fire codes.

- Consider implementing an infant security tag or abduction alarm system.

As care providers for both mothers and infants, nurses are in an excellent position to help ensure the safety and security of the care environment and use of security mechanisms as intended. Strategies nurses can use to help prevent infant abductions follow.

Prevention Strategies

Participate on multidisciplinary teams to develop and implement or improve infant security policy and procedures. Nurses should participate on teams addressing access control policies and procedures. Their input into how to secure entry points, including access to doors for visitors and staff, can be critical. Nurses working in areas where infants and mothers receive care are well equipped to join other disciplines, such as risk management, building security, and maintenance, to review the security of means of access to and egress from the units. The nursing staff needs to be involved in selecting security equipment and in the piloting of new devices.

Help ensure monitoring of entry and exit points and functioning of doors and alarms. People who want to accomplish something can be both inventive and creative in developing ways to "get around the system." For example, staff frequently encounter novel door wedges and holding devices that compromise the security of entry and exit points. On a routine basis, nurses can ask appropriate staff to manually test doors for compromising factors and check doors with alarms to ensure that alarms are functioning. All faulty doors or alarms should be reported and no devices or alarms should ever be disabled.

Check security devices used on mothers and infants. Reliance on security tags and other devices can, at times, create a false sense of security. Nurses can verify that devices used on the infant and mother are working. Whenever security equipment such as security clamps are used to identify/protect the infant, they must be thoroughly tested for function not only on purchase but on a regular basis thereafter. Nurses can help to ensure that all devices are included in the organization's equipment maintenance plan.

Check the identification of baby and parents whenever the baby is passed to a parent or returned to the nursery from a parent. It is critical that the identification is verified and accurate. Too often the wrist and ankle bands on the infant come off and are pinned to the bassinet. When any identification band comes off, new banding should be performed with the mother and father/significant other and in the presence of a witness. When babies spend time in the nursery as well as in the mother's room, establish a tracking system to document where the infant is at all times.

Know what the experts recommend in the area of physical security. Nurses familiar with physical security guidelines proposed by the NCMEC can advocate for their organization's adherence to the guidelines. These appear as Sidebar 5-2, page 64.

Root Cause 2: Inadequate Patient Education

Sentinel Event Example: Inadequate Care Recipient Education. *A woman enters a hospital and provides a staff member at the information desk with the name and room number of a woman who has recently given birth, whom she indicates she will be visiting. She is given a visitor's pass. The visitor proceeds to the maternal care/newborn nursery unit and finds the mother's room, which she enters. The visitor befriends the mother and spends a couple of hours talking with her while the new mother awaits her husband's arrival. Needing to use the bathroom, the mother asks the visitor to hold her baby, while she is in the bathroom. When the mother emerges a few minutes later, the visitor and baby are gone.*

This example illustrates the effects of inadequate staff and care recipient education, the

SIDEBAR 5-2. GUIDELINES FOR PHYSICAL SECURITY

■ Every health care facility must develop a written assessment of the risk potential for an infant abduction.

■ Install alarms, preferably with time-delay locks, on all stairwell and exit doors leading to/from or in close proximity to the maternity, nursery, neonatal-intensive-care, and pediatrics units. Establish a policy of responding to alarms and instruct responsible staff to silence and reset an activated alarm only after direct observation of the stairwell or exit and the person using it. The alarm system should never be disabled.

■ All nursery doors must have self-closing hardware, remain locked at all times, and a staff member should be present at all times when an infant is in the nursery.

■ Install a security-camera system (using time-lapse loop tape such as those employed in banks) or digital-recording technology to monitor activity in the halls of the maternity and the pediatrics floors. The cameras should be placed in strategic spots at the entrance of the unit to cover the nursery, hallway, stairwells, elevators and adjusted at an angle to capture an abductor's full face. Videotape recorders need to be functional and someone needs to be responsible for changing tapes daily. Retain videotapes for a minimum of seven days before reusing.

■ Take particular care to position one camera that will capture the faces of all persons using any entrance to the maternal-child-care unit.

Source: Rabun JB: *For Healthcare Professionals: Guidelines on Prevention of and Response to Infant Abductions—Sixth Edition.* Arlington, VA: National Center for Missing & Exploited Children, Mar 2000, pp 18–20. Used with permission.

latter of which is our focus here. The mother was not properly educated about the risk of giving her infant to someone without proper staff identification. Nurses are involved in providing care recipient and family education that promotes and maintains health, fosters care, and improves outcomes. Education should be presented in ways that are understandable to those receiving them, taking into account literacy, educational levels, and language, among other factors. Education should also be interactive so that nursing staff can ensure that the information is understood. Education includes information about care recipient responsibilities in the care recipient's care area, which again, nurses generally provide.

Mothers and families need to be educated on the precautions that the organization has taken with the design of the unit and why. They need to be aware that all remote exits are alarmed and locked from the outside to prevent access. They need to know that unauthorized entry on the unit by persons without a pass or after visit-

ing hours without authorization is prohibited. They should be informed that their newborn will be banded along with the mother in the delivery room, that the infant will have two matching bands—one on the wrist and one on the ankle. In some organizations, the infant will also have an umbilical clamp with a sensor that would sound an alarm should anyone attempt to take the infant off the unit.

The mother and families also need to be educated on how to recognize unit nurses, such as by special identification badges with pictures of the nurse, specific colored uniforms, and so forth. The mothers need to know that they should not give their babies to anyone not identified as one of "their" nurses. They need to know the name of their nurse on each shift. If there is any question regarding the nurse or someone on the unit, the mother or her family should notify their nurse or the charge nurse immediately. Experts recommend that staff who are allowed to take babies from mothers or to the nursery wear a highly visible photograph identification badge. "This becomes a baby O.K. hall pass," says Rabun.[4] Colling has seen hospitals use clever informational reminders such as placing stickers on bathroom doors or tent cards on tables in the postpartum room.

After educating mothers and families about which staff members they can release their baby to, mothers sign a form to acknowledge that organization staff provided this information. NCMEC's summary of educational content that hospital personnel can provide parents to help prevent abduction of infants while in health care facilities appears as Sidebar 5-3, page 66.

To help prevent both infant abductions and discharge to wrong family sentinel events, some organizations have developed programs "partnering" with parents. Taught by nurses, and sometimes presented jointly with other community agencies, police, at churches, and community events, this program helps parents protect their child throughout the child's most vulnerable years. Topics include how to help deter abduction in the hospital and after discharge, community resources to assist in fingerprinting children and updating child IDs, tips on infant protection in malls, stores, and other topics.

Prevention Strategies

Effectively educate mothers and their families about abduction risks. New parents generally experience anxiety about their infants. Nurses need to teach in a manner that will not scare the mothers and families but instead, communicate a caring concern for the safety and well being of their infants and children. Enhanced parent education concerning abduction risks and parent responsibility for reducing risk as well as timely assessment of the parents' level of understanding are critical to the reduction of abduction risk.

Regularly reinforce education. Because new parents can easily be overwhelmed by the presence of staff, visitors, and care concerns, nurses can take an active role in reminding them of security precautions.

Root Cause 3: Insufficient Staff Orientation, Training, Competence, or Credentialing or Insufficient Staffing Levels

"Near Miss" Example: Insufficient Staff Training and Competence Assessment. *In a large metropolitan hospital, five obstetrical discharges are scheduled for a Saturday morning. Because the unit is very busy, the nursing supervisor "pulls" a cross-trained nurse to help with the discharges. One mother is ready for discharge when the pulled nurse arrives on the unit. The nurse goes to the nursery and wraps "baby boy Smith" in the blanket the mother gave her. The nurse checks the baby's and mother's arm-bands. Both indicate "Smith." When the nurse brings the baby to the mother, the mother notices that the infant has a birth mark on his face which was not previously there. The mother notifies the charge nurse that this is not her baby. In fact, two "baby boy Smiths" are ready for discharge that morning and the cross-trained nurse had not checked the baby's identification numbers with the mother's numbers on the arm bands.*

"Near Miss" Example: Insufficient Staff Training and Insufficient Staffing Levels. *A hospital's infant security management plan was developed and implemented without the participation of the organization's nursing and medical staffs. Staff and physician education about the plan was minimal at best, and there was no follow up to assure competence. Staff generally was not aware of how breaches of the plan could increase the risk of infant abduction from the labor, delivery, and post-partum care areas. The policy involved locked doors on the unit and the use of a code or badge entry. The medical staff felt that badge entry was too time-consuming and could delay their care to obstetrical patients, especially when a delivery or a "crash C-section" was needed in a hurry. Staff modified the plan to allow physicians to circumvent the badge entry. Both nursing and medical staff felt that the plan was not "user friendly" and that families might not like being locked in or out. Dissatisfaction notwithstanding, the staff oriented mothers to the infant security system upon admission to the unit.*

A woman is admitted to the unit in active labor during a very busy time on the unit. There have been an unusual number of deliveries in the past 48 hours and the nursing staff has worked many extra hours. The admitting nurse assesses the mother to determine

SIDEBAR 5-3. WHAT PARENTS NEED TO KNOW

Hospital personnel should remind parents, in a warm and comforting way, of the measures they should take to provide maximum child protection. The guidelines listed below provide good, sound parenting techniques that can also help prevent abduction of infants while in the healthcare facility where the child was born.

1. At some point before the birth of your baby, investigate security procedures at the facility where you plan to give birth to your baby and request a copy of the facility's written guidelines on procedures for "special care" and security procedures in the maternity ward. Know all of the facility's procedures that are in place to safeguard your infant while staying in that facility.

2. While it is normal for new parents to be anxious, being deliberately watchful over the newborn infant is of paramount importance.

3. Never leave your infant out of your direct line-of-sight even when you go to the bathroom or take a nap. If you leave the room or plan to go to sleep, alert the nurses to take the infant back to the nursery or have a family member watch the baby. When possible, keep the infant's bassinet on the side of your bed that is away from the door(s) leading out of the room.

4. After admission to the facility, ask about hospital protocols concerning the routine nursery procedures, feeding and visitation hours, and security measures.

5. Do not give your infant to anyone without properly verified hospital identification. Find out what additional or special identification is being worn to further identify those hospital personnel who have authority to handle the infant.

6. Become familiar with the hospital staff who work in the maternity unit. During short stays in the hospital, ask to be introduced to the nurse assigned to you and your infant.

7. Question unfamiliar persons entering your room or inquiring about your infant—even if they are in hospital attire or seem to have a reason for being there. Alert the nurses' station immediately.

8. Determine where your infant will be when taken for tests, and how long the tests will take. Find out who has authorized the tests. If you are uncomfortable with anyone who requests to take your baby or unable to clarify what testing is being done or why your baby is being taken from your room, it is appropriate to go with your baby to observe the procedure.

9. For your records to take home, have at least one color photograph of your infant (full, front-face view) taken and compile a complete written description of your infant including hair and eye color, length, weight, date of birth, and specific physical attributes.

10. At some point after the birth of your baby, but before discharge from the facility, request a set of written guidelines on the procedures for any follow-up care extended by the facility that will be scheduled to take place in your home. Do not allow anyone into your home who says that he or she is affiliated with the facility without properly verified hospital identification. Find out what additional or special identification is being worn to further identify those staff members who have authority to enter your home.

11. Consider the risk you may be taking when permitting your infant's birth announcement to be published in the newspaper or online. Birth announcements should never include the family's home address and should be limited to the parents' surname(s).

Source: Rabun JB: *For Healthcare Professionals: Guidelines on Prevention of and Response to Infant Abductions—Sixth Edition.* Arlington, VA: National Center for Missing & Exploited Children, Mar 2000, pp 43–44. Used with permission.

the stage of labor but, because of the delivery of another baby which she must attend to, the nurse decides to complete the woman's orientation to the unit after that delivery. She is admitted to the birthing room, where two other women are in active labor.

Meanwhile, in the delivery room, yet another woman is delivering her baby. The charge nurse calls the supervisor to request extra staff due to the high level of activity in the labor and delivery rooms. The supervisor evaluates this request and decides to provide assistance herself until after the delivery, at which point, she feels that the staff will be able to care for all of the patients in labor.

The delivery occurs immediately before a change of shift in the nurse staffing. Nurses on duty have already worked a 12-hour shift. The nurse who admitted this woman goes home, forgetting to tell the next shift of nurses that the woman needs to be oriented to the infant security system.

The woman delivers her baby approximately two hours later and is returned to the postpartum unit with her newborn. Her family visits and she falls asleep shortly thereafter with her baby beside her in a bassinet. On awakening, she looks in the bassinet and notices that her baby is not there. The woman calls the nurse and asks that her baby be brought back to her room. The nurse tells her that the baby is not in the nursery, calls the desk, and reports the baby missing. The baby is found with the father in the hospital lobby. He had brought the newborn down to show him off to other family members.

These examples illustrates numerous failures, including failure to ensure adequate staff orientation, training, and competence, failure to ensure an adequate staffing level, and inadequate communication among caregivers. The first two failures are discussed here; the third failure is addressed in the next section.

All personnel must be oriented to and educated about the environment of care and possess the knowledge and skills to perform their responsibilities in this environment. Particular attention should be given to security-sensitive areas such as the obstetrical and pediatric areas. Directors provide for orientation, in-service training, and continuing education of all persons in the

department. An orientation process provides initial job training and information key to assessing the staff's ability to fulfill specified responsibilities. Continuing in-services, educational sessions, hospital newsletters, town hall meetings, and staff meetings are a number of possible means of keeping nurses and others informed of relevant changes and updates following initial training. Leaders must ensure that staff competence is assessed on a regular basis. The floating nurse in the first example was not competent in the organization's infant-mother identification procedures.

Through orientation, training, and ongoing assessment, staff learn how to properly implement an organization's security plan. The nurse staff needs to be oriented to any new policies, procedures, protocols, or equipment used in their care units. Nursing staff also must receive information on prevention procedures and the critical incident response plan. Both physicians and nurses in the second example did not understand how their actions compromised the organization's security plan. Physicians bypassed the badge entry system; nurses did not complete education in a timely fashion. Personnel were not informed about security in sensitive areas and therefore were obstructing the design of the security plan. Because nursing and medical staff were not involved in the development of the security plan, their understanding and "buy in" were lacking.

If cross-trained staff is used to provide adequate staffing on the unit, leaders must ensure that the staff is knowledgeable about current and new organization policies and protocols. Leaders should encourage use of the "buddy" system, that is, pairing a cross-trained nurse with a regular obstetrical/nursery nurse for as long a period of time as possible. Regular nursing staff can convey the message, "If in doubt, please ask questions." Some organizations appoint floating nurses only to assignments that they would perform on their regular unit. In this scenario, regular unit nurses care for those individuals that require skills used specifically on the obstetrical/nursery unit, such as the banding of babies, deliveries, discharges, and so forth. A quick review sheet, including specific information that floating nurses may not be as familiar with, can be a helpful tool.

In order to ensure discharge to the right family, organizations must have a formal policy and procedure for proper infant identification. Identification needs to be verified by the nurse not by just name, as there may be more than one infant with the same last name, but also by identification number. If a third party has a band, it should be checked with the mother and infant. Many organizations are now using security clamps (umbilical clamps) on infants. If these security clamps also contain an identification number, they should be part of the identification process. Other organizations are using a bar coding system to verify infant and parent identity.

Leaders must ensure an adequate number of staff members whose qualifications are consistent with job responsibilities to meet care recipient needs. Leaders in the hospital profiled in the second example did not ensure appropriate staffing levels. With adequate staffing, the time to orient the mother would have been available.

Leadership and human resources staff identify the methodology for adequate staffing based on the needs of the care recipient. Care areas that increase census rapidly require additional skill and ingenuity to create staffing patterns that meet needs. Many hospitals have nursing on-call lists, supplemental staff, and cross-trained staff to address staffing needs during a fluctuating census.

Prevention Strategies

Increase knowledge of risk factors for infant abduction and discharge to wrong family. Nurses need to be educated not only regarding the organization's philosophy, policy and procedure related to preventing infant abductions or release to the wrong families or wrong family members, but also what is cited in current literature and required by regulatory bodies. Too often, literature is sent to the unit manager, put in a folder or file cabinet and not distributed to unit nurses. Leaders must support the continuing education of nurses concerning risk factors for infant abduction and discharge to wrong family. Monographs and articles appearing in the professional literature (including *Sentinel Event Alerts*) and the news media can be distributed to

all nurses and discussed at unit meetings. Guest speakers and seminars related to the early identification of risk factors and prevention of infant abduction and discharge to the wrong family provide an excellent means to enhance nursing knowledge and skills.

Know and adhere to the security/safety plan, policies, and procedures. Nurses must feel comfortable about their ability to describe, demonstrate, and implement the organization's plan and processes for minimizing security risks, emergency procedures for security incidents, and reporting procedures for security incidents involving care recipients, visitors, personnel, and property. Participating in abduction drills conducted periodically by the health care organization can help to give nurses—as well as all staff—confidence in their ability to react properly in a real abduction. They also must follow organization policies and procedures for ensuring the proper identification of the mother and baby. For example, before a baby is discharged, nurses must check the bands/clamps carefully not only for the name of baby and mother but also the identification number. If the organization has a discharge checklist, nurses should use it at the time of discharge rather than filling it in later. Asking the mother to examine the infant to be sure that it is her baby and then have her sign the checklist can help prevent discharge to wrong family sentinel events.

Be familiar with available technology and use it properly. Many new and innovative security devices are on the market. However, if the nurse is unfamiliar with them, does not use them as intended, or does not report failures, the full security benefits will not be realized. Instances when an umbilical security clamp has come off and has been pinned or tapped to the bassinet have been cited in numerous organizations. This practice defeats the purpose of the clamp. Nurses must be an integral part of any teams evaluating new security technology.

Inform supervisor of unsafe staffing practices. As mentioned in earlier chapters, nurses should use the communication channels established in their organizations to express concern about unsafe staffing levels or practices that could result in an infant abduction or discharge to wrong family.

Root Cause 4: Communication or Information-related Failure

Communication and coordination among caregivers are critical to the prevention of infant abductions and release to wrong families. Inadequate communication among nursing staff members contributed to the near miss events described under Root Cause 3. Relevant information regarding the status of the woman's education about the organization's infant security program was not passed along to nursing staff members on the next shift. It is imperative that caregivers and care recipients communicate relevant information at all times. The change of shifts is often a hectic time. However, it is extremely important that the next shift be informed of any possible safety or security concerns. Communication is imperative, for example, if a security device such as an umbilical clamp, is not working or not secured properly, if infant/family wrist and ankle bands come off, or the banding was not completed per organization policy.

Prevention Strategies

Ensure thorough communication and use documentation to enhance the transfer of relevant information. Nurses as well as other staff must not rely on verbal communication alone. Written documentation such as checklists, notes, and reports is necessary to avoid poor health care outcomes.

Communicate with unfamiliar persons on the unit and be assertive in validating their legitimate presence. Check identification of all visitors. Alert supervisor and take appropriate actions when visitors exhibit unusual behavior. Nurses need to be aware of individuals who visit nursery, postpartum, and pediatric areas and must follow organization security and safety procedures and protocols. Unauthorized visitors or staff cannot be allowed. This may be hard for some staff to accept. They may feel torn between wanting to provide a customer-friendly environment and

yet concerned for the safety and well-being of their care recipients. There is often a great deal of pressure to "make just this one exception." Colling recommends that nurses introduce themselves to visitors or staff they don't know and be assertive when seeing strangers in corridors, including individuals who appear to be staff members but are unfamiliar to the nurse.[4] Nursing staff must be continuously alert for any unusual behaviors of visitors on the unit and need to be able to report any suspicious behavior without fear of retribution. All concerns regarding visitors or potential security problems must be reported immediately.

Advocate for the organization to discontinue providing birth notices to local newspapers. Providing birth notices to local newspapers used to be standard practice by organizations, but is not as regularly seen today. Publication of information regarding infant births increases the risk of infant abduction. If the organization continues to provide birth information to the media, nursing staff can communicate concern through the organization's established channels.

NCMEC's guidelines[1] on the prevention of and response to infant abductions provide additional security strategies and protocols that support and enhance the Joint Commission's standards on security issues. A partial list of proactive steps organization leaders can take to reduce the risk of infant abductions appears as Sidebar 5-4, page 70.

Concluding Comments

Infant abductions or release to the wrong families are sentinel events with particularly devastating impact. Nurses can take a proactive approach to reducing the risk of such sentinel events. Strategies include helping to ensure: a safe environment of care, properly functioning and used security equipment, high quality patient and family education, and thorough training, competence assessment, and caregiver communication.

SIDEBAR 5-4. PROACTIVE PREVENTIVE MEASURES

- Develop a written proactive prevention plan.
- Immediately after birth of infant, attach identically numbered ID bands to infant (two bands), mother (one band), and father or significant other (one band), when appropriate.
- Prior to removal of newborn from birthing room, footprint the baby, take color photo, perform/record full physical assessment, and note all these items in the baby's medical chart. Store a sample of the infant's cord blood until at least one day after the infant's discharge.
- Require all health care personnel to wear up-to-date, conspicuous, color photo ID badges; personnel in direct contact with infants should wear a second form of unique identification (for example, pink background on badge).
- Distribute prevention guidelines to parents in childbirth classes, on preadmission tours, upon admission, and at postpartum instruction.
- Train staff in protecting infants from abduction.
- To safeguard transportation of infants within the facility, ensure that infants are only transported by authorized staff, never left in the hallway without direct supervision, taken to mothers one at a time, and always pushed in bassinets rather than carried.
- Always place infants in direct, line-of-sight supervision either by a responsible staff member, the mother, or other family member/close friend so designated by the mother. Address the procedure to be followed when the baby is with the mother and she needs to go to sleep or to the bathroom and/or is sedated.
- Do not post the mother's or infant's full name where it will be visible to visitors.
- Establish an access-control policy for the nursing unit, including nursery, maternity, neonatal intensive care, and pediatrics.
- Instruct facility personnel at the front lobby or entrance to any of these units to ask visitors which mother they are visiting and for how long. If no name is known or given, decline admission and alert appropriate parties.
- Require the person taking the infant home from the facility to show his or her ID wristband; match the band with those worn by the infant.
- Never divulge the home address or other unique information in public birth announcements (which put the infant at risk after discharge).

Source: Rabun JB: *For Healthcare Professionals: Guidelines on Prevention of and Response to Infant Abductions—Sixth Edition.* Arlington, VA: National Center for Missing & Exploited Children, Mar 2000. Used with permission.

References

1. National Center for Missing & Exploited Children: Press Release: Coordinated response to infant abductions from healthcare facilities pays off, Jan 6, 2000.

2. Rabun JB: *For Healthcare Professionals: Guidelines on Prevention of and Response to Infant Abductions—Sixth Edition.* Arlington, VA: National Center for Missing & Exploited Children, Mar 2000, p 3. Web site: *www.missingkids.org.*

3. Rabun JB (2000), p 7.

4. Joint Commission: Infant abductions: Preventing future occurrences. *Sentinel Event Alert* Issue 9, Apr 9, 1999.

Chapter 6:

Preventing Serious Injury or Death in Physical Restraint

Violence by individuals receiving care against fellow care recipients, health care staff, and visitors represents a problem in all health care facilities, particularly those providing behavioral health services. Falls by individuals receiving care also present a problem in all facilities and home care. Fall prevention and aggression often lead to restraint use. Wandering, agitation, confusion, and aggressive outbursts by individuals receiving care are frequently cited reasons for the use of physical restraint.

Physical restraint is dangerous. When used improperly, it can lead to death or serious injury. The best way to avoid such risk is to *not* use physical restraint. At times, however, physical restraint may be the only possible alternative to prevent harm to the individual or other persons or to ensure a safe treatment environment when other interventions are not effective or appropriate.

Restraint Defined

The Joint Commission defines a *physical restraint* as any method of physically restricting a person's freedom of movement, physical activity, and normal access to the body.[1] This encompasses many physical devices, such as wrist restraints, jacket vests, and mitts, as well as physical procedures such as therapeutic or protective holds. For purposes of this discussion, restraint differs from medical immobilization, such as body restraint during surgery, arm restraint during intravenous administration, and temporary physical restraint before administration of electroconvulsive therapy.[2] These are considered a regular part of such procedures. In long term care organizations, *restraint* is

defined as any method (chemical* or physical) of restricting a resident's freedom of movement, including seclusion, physical activity, or normal access to his or her body that

1. is not a usual and customary part of a medical diagnostic or treatment procedure to which the resident or his or her legal representative has consented;

2. is not indicated to treat the resident's medical condition or symptoms; or

3. does not promote the resident's independent functioning.[2]

Cause for Concern

The FDA estimates that at least 100 deaths result each year from improper use of restraint devices.[3] The actual number of deaths may very well be higher. Although the Safe Medical Devices Act of 1990 requires all hospitals, nursing homes, and acute care facilities to report deaths related to the use of any medical device to the FDA and the manufacturer, many restraint-related deaths may never have been reported anywhere, particularly those involving protective holds. In October 1998, a series of articles appearing in *The Hartford Courant* reported on deaths following use of physical restraint in behavioral health care facilities. A 50-state survey conducted by the Connecticut newspaper revealed at least 142 deaths in the past decade connected with the use of physical restraint or seclusion.[4] Another survey conducted for the

---

* For the purposes of this chapter, sentinel events resulting from the use of chemical restraints are not considered a restraint-related sentinel event, but rather, a medication-related sentinel event. These are covered in Chapter 2.

SIDEBAR 6-1. FACTORS THAT MAY CONTRIBUTE TO AN INCREASED RISK OF RESTRAINT-RELATED DEATH

Joint Commission analysis identified the following factors that may contribute to an increased risk of death. These include restraining an individual

■ who smokes;

■ with deformities that preclude the proper application of a restraining device (especially vest restraints);

■ in the supine position (may predispose the individual to aspiration);

■ in the prone position (may predispose the individual to suffocation); and

■ in a room that is not under continuous observation by staff.

Source: Joint Commission: Preventing restraint deaths. *Sentinel Event Alert* Issue 8, Nov 18, 1998.

---

newspaper by a research specialist at the Harvard Center for Risk Analysis estimated that 50 to 150 such deaths may occur each year.

Data from the Joint Commission's Sentinel Event database indicate that restraint-related deaths and injuries represent 4.5% of all sentinel events reviewed by the Joint Commission between January 1995 and January 2001. Of the deaths, the majority occurred in psychiatric hospitals, followed by general hospitals, and long term care facilities. In 40% of the cases cited in the Joint Commission's *Sentinel Event Alert,* the cause of death was asphyxiation.[5] Asphyxiation was related to factors such as

■ putting excessive weight on the back of the individual in a prone position;

■ placing a towel or sheet over the individual's head to protect against spitting or biting; or

■ obstructing the airway when pulling the individual's arm across the neck area.

The remaining deaths were caused by strangulation, cardiac arrest, or fire. All the victims of strangulation death were elderly individuals who had been placed in a vest restraint. All the victims of death by fire were males who were attempting to smoke or use a cigarette lighter to burn off the restraint. Two-point, four-point or five-point restraints were used on extremities in 40% of the cases related to restraint deaths. A therapeutic hold was used in 30% of the cases, a restraint vest was used in 20%, and a

waist restraint was used in 10% of the cases. Factors identified by Joint Commission staff that may contribute to an increased risk of deaths appear in Sidebar 6-1, above.

Root Causes and Prevention Strategies

A review of the literature indicates that organizations with a lower incidence of violence and of restraint and seclusion use share several key attributes. These appear in Sidebar 6-2, page 73.

Organizations that experienced a sentinel event related to restraint use reviewed by the Joint Commission identified the following root causes[5]:

■ *Staffing issues, including insufficient staff orientation, training, competence assessment, or credentialing or insufficient staffing levels;*

■ *Unsafe equipment or equipment use,* such as: use of split side rails without side rail protectors; use of two-point rather than four-point restraints; use of a high-neck vest; incorrect application of a restraining device; or a monitor or an alarm not working or not being used when appropriate;

■ *Lack of adequate observation procedures or practices;*

■ *Inadequate assessment,* including incomplete examination of the individual to identify contraband, such as matches; and

---

SIDEBAR 6-2. KEY ATTRIBUTES OF ORGANIZATIONS WITH A LOWER INCIDENCE OF VIOLENCE AND RESTRAINT AND SECLUSION USE

- Leaders clearly advocate a treatment philosophy;

- Individuals at risk for violence are identified through assessment on admission to the facility or program;

- Staff is well-trained in aggression management;

- Staff practices encourage maximum use of behavioral modification and de-escalation techniques and minimal use of restraint and seclusion;

- Increased activities for individuals correlate with decreased usage rates of restraints and seclusion;

- The need for restraint or seclusion is based on an evaluation of the individual case and situation; and

- The staff follow guidelines or protocols when restraint or seclusion is indicated.

Source: Joint Commission: *Preventing Adverse Events in Behavioral Health Care: A Systems Approach to Sentinel Events.* Oakbrook Terrace, IL: Joint Commission on Accreditation of Healthcare Organizations, 1999.

- *Inadequate care planning,* such as alternatives to restraints not fully considered, restraints used as punishment, and inappropriate room or unit assignment.

More than 90% of the organizations cited insufficient staff orientation and training as a root cause; 80% cited equipment-related factors; and 65% cited lack of care recipient observation procedures or practices. Figure 6-1, page 74, provides a graphic look at the frequency of each type of root cause. A closer look at each root cause will help to identify strategies nurses can use to reduce the likelihood of restraint-related deaths and injuries.

Root Cause 1: Insufficient Staff Orientation, Training, Competence Assessment, or Credentialing

Sentinel Event Example: Insufficient Orientation. *A temporary staff member, who normally works in the newborn nursery of the obstetrics area, is assigned to work in a surgical area where most care recipients are over the age of 75. The staff member is not knowledgeable about the effects of anesthesia on the elderly or selection and application of physical restraint.*

After working on the unit for less than an hour, the temporary staff member sees one post surgical patient attempting to climb over his bed rails. The staff

member applies the first type of physical restraint that he can find (a vest), without calling the individual's physician for an order. He then continues to care for other individuals, neglecting to report use of the vest to the charge nurse.

When the man's son arrives 45 minutes later to visit his father, recovering from a routine appendectomy, he finds his father hanging from the restraint which is attached to the bed rail. His father is blue, cold and has only a faint pulse. A code is called and staff attempt to revive the man. He is placed on a ventilator and admitted to the intensive care unit, but dies one hour later.

Organization leaders must ensure that an orientation process provides initial job training and that each staff member's ability to meet the performance expectations stated in his or her job description are assessed *before* the staff member provides direct care. During general staff orientation, each staff member must receive basic information regarding restraint use in the organization and alternatives to physical restraint. Clinical staff members then receive more in-depth information and training and must demonstrate their competence in restraint application and care of the individual in restraints before providing care. Competence assessment can best be accomplished through both written testing and practical application in

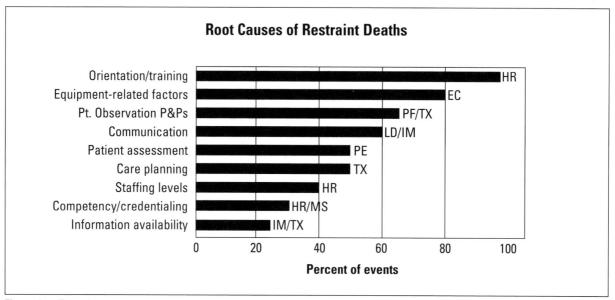

Figure 6-1. *This chart illustrates the percentage of causes at the root of restraint-related deaths reported to the Joint Commission between January 1995 and January 2001.*

the education setting before allowing the individual to apply restraints in the clinical setting.

Staff from all shifts as well as part-time and per diem individuals must be included in restraint use orientation, training, and competence assessment programs. Medical, nursing and allied health students, physicians, nurses, nursing assistants, therapists, and others who may also need to be educated and assessed on restraint policies and procedures should not be overlooked. New staff, agency staff, or staff floated from another area who are not familiar with care recipients or who are not regularly assigned to the unit may cause injury as illustrated in the previous example. Reassessment of competence must occur regularly, as defined by the organization. Because restraint use is a high-risk area and staff may not frequently use restraint, annual competence assessment is warranted.

Staffing adequacy is vital in organizations in which restraint is used and more so if the use of restraint is to be minimized. Nursing staffing numbers may need to be adjusted to make allocations for the necessary numbers of clinical staff to provide care and frequently assess the condition of individuals in restraint. Nursing supervisors must identify whether more staff is required in specific areas due to restraint use. All organizations should have adequate numbers

of staff to identify alternatives to restraint and seclusion use or, if unavoidable, to quickly, effectively, and safely apply restraint or assist the individual into a seclusion area. Injury to staff and care recipients can occur when an adequate number of trained staff members are not available to apply restraint and monitor individuals in restraint.

Prevention Strategies

Know the alternatives. The nursing literature is full of information related to psychosocial, physiologic, environmental, and pharmaco-therapeutic interventions that can be used appropriately and effectively instead of physical restraint. For example, the use of bed, chair, or door alarms are good alternatives to physical restraint for care recipients who may wander. Proper pain assessment and management may be the issue for some individuals. Increased use of non-medication alternatives, such as massage therapy, can increase the individual's comfort without increasing symptoms such as mental confusion that could increase the apparent need for restraint use. In some cases, reduced dosages of pain medication can be administered, which also will decrease hypnotic side effects, drowsiness, and mental confusion. Some organizations also use family members or properly trained "sitters" to stay with the individual as an alternative to restraint.

SIDEBAR 6-3. RESTRAINT ALTERNATIVES

- Use active listening, verbal de-escalation and other anger management techniques.

- Provide quiet areas or rooms for use when individuals are angry or upset. Rooms equipped with punching bags or treadmills let care recipients work off energy without threatening others.

- Teach social skills to correct maladaptive behavior.

- Use motivational therapy, such as a "token economy," for assaultive individuals. A *token economy* is a motivational behavioral treatment that offers incentives for individuals to engage in desirable, functional behaviors, and decrease the frequency of undesirable, assaultive behaviors that lead to the use of restraint and seclusion.

- Ensure proper pain management, toileting program, and nutritional care to relieve any discomfort experienced by care recipients.

- Provide regular exercise programs to increase care recipient mobility and muscle strength. Consider enlisting a recreational, physical, or occupational therapist to lead the sessions.

- Increase physical and mental exercise programs for restless individuals. Keep cognitively impaired persons busy.

- Equip rooms with alternative types of seating, such as recliners or seats with adaptive cushions, that enable care recipients to maintain their center of gravity while sitting.

- Use wrist, bed, or chair alarms that are sensitive to movement or pressure and door alarms that alert staff to individuals who are moving about without supervision.

- Post cues, such as stop signs, at exits to remind care recipients where they can and cannot go in the facility.

- Provide a safe enclosed area for individuals who wander.

- Design safe environments with few obstructions but plenty of visual stimulation (for example, posters and other wall hangings) to encourage exploration.

- Create a homelike familiar atmosphere in rooms of those who are agitated, confused, or aggressive. Family photographs or a favorite afghan or blanket can have a calming effect.

- Encourage volunteers and family members to provide companionship. Provide pet therapy, if possible.

- Plan activities to occupy individuals who are restless at night or who suffer from insomnia. Quiet games, headphones for listening to audiotapes, and relaxation techniques can help.

- Limit accessibility to life-support lines. If tube feedings are necessary, consider using a percutaneous endoscopic gastrostomy tube. This can easily be hidden by clothing, and individuals rarely disrupt it.

Source: Abstracted from Joint Commission: *Reducing Restraint Use in the Acute Care Environment.* Oakbrook Terrace, IL: Joint Commission on Accreditation of Healthcare Organizations, 1998.

Sidebar 6-3, above, provides numerous other examples of alternatives to restraint. Nurses need to remain current with alternatives suggested in the literature. Articles from recent literature can be retained in a notebook on the nursing unit. Nurses can initial each article after reading it. Staff meetings can also include discussion of new trends reported in the literature as well as new rules and regulations issued by regulatory bodies. Training and in-service sessions can provide nurses with a wealth of restraint alternatives.

Ensure personal competence in restraint use and monitoring and help ensure competence of those working with you. Nurses must feel comfortable about their knowledge of restraint alternatives, their ability to assess the need for restraint and to apply restraint safely, and their skill in monitoring and assessing the individual in restraint. If they do not feel well-trained and competent, they should let their supervisor know that they need more training and supervision. Nurses should not assume that those working around them have been properly educated or trained in restraint use. Talking with students and other staff members about restraint use can indicate if the person has had the training and possesses the skills to use restraints competently and appropriately. Supervisors can be notified about apparent deficiencies.

Help to ensure proper orders for restraint use. Physicians and licensed independent practitioners (LIPs) need to be properly knowledgeable about the theory of physical restraint use, the need to limit use to a specific short duration. They also must know how to direct staff to use restraints through the orders the physicians provide. Often physicians or LIPs will write "restrain as needed" or use physical restraint "prn." Joint Commission standards and laws in most states prohibit nursing staff from following such orders. The order needs to be time limited, specific as to the type of device used, and the reason for the device's use. Orders may be given to clinical staff only after all reasonable alternatives have been tried and failed and documentation of attempts and failures appears in the clinical record. Nurses can help ensure that physician orders are appropriate and documented properly.

Inform supervisor of unsafe staffing levels. Recommend a revised staffing model. See discussion in previous chapters (pages 43, 53, and 65). As appropriate, nurses may wish to recommend the development of a pool of trained, competent volunteers who can "sit" with those at risk for restraint use, provide one-on-one observation while also reading to the individual, providing music therapy, aroma therapy, or other therapies.

Root Cause 2: Unsafe Equipment or Environment or Unsafe Equipment Use

"Near Miss" Example: Improper Use of Equipment.
An individual receiving residential care in a facility

for the developmentally delayed and physically challenged has a customized electric wheel chair that is specially fitted to his physical condition. The wheelchair lets the man be somewhat mobile while seated properly and safely without using restraints. As scheduled, the wheelchair is sent out for repair and replacement of some of the fitted cushions. The man receives a "loaner" chair which is not designed to meet his positioning and mobility needs. During this time, staff members do what they can to provide for the man's mobility, comfort, and safety. One staff member applies a waist-type restraining device to help the man remain in an upright position while in the wheelchair. However, instead of applying the device around the waist as it is intended to be used, the staff member applies it around the man's chest and under both arms. The man twists out of the proper position rather quickly. When the staff member returns twenty minutes later to check the man, he has large red areas under both arms and across the front of his neck. These later turn into huge purple bruises. Fortunately, the improperly applied restraint did not obstruct the man's airway.

Prevention strategies for this root cause are closely related to those for the first root cause related to staff training and assessment. A properly trained nurse recognizes unsafe equipment and knows how to use safe equipment effectively and appropriately. Selecting the wrong type of restraint for a particular individual's needs, putting a restraint on backwards or upside down, or using the wrong size increases the likelihood of injury or death. For example, injury can occur when the care recipient's head is elevated while a restraint device is tied to the stationary part of the bed frame.

A sound equipment maintenance program requires inspection and testing of all restraint equipment before use. A preventive maintenance program reassesses the safety of equipment at specified intervals throughout the year, as per organization policy and manufacturer guidelines.

Prevention Strategies

Select safe equipment and use equipment safely. Nursing staff often play a key role in selecting, purchasing, and applying restraint devices. The FDA advises health care staff to follow the directions provided by the device's manufacturer to[4]

- select the type of restraint recommended for the individual's condition;
- use the correct size for the individual's weight and height;
- note the front and back of the restraint and apply correctly;
- tie knots that can be released quickly;
- secure bed restraints to the bed springs or frame, never to the mattress or bed rails. With an adjustable bed, secure the restraints to the parts of the bed that move with the individual.

Many experts recommend discontinuing the use of high-risk equipment such as the high vest, waist restraint devices, and unprotected split side rails.[5] Even with proper use of safe devices, device failures occur. For example, a restraint device under stress might break away or rip. Finally, nurses must monitor all individuals in restraint to ensure their continued safety.

Help to ensure a safe environment of care. A safe care environment helps to reduce the use of restraint. Nurses can remove obstacles that impede an individual's movement, place objects and furniture in familiar places, lower beds, place non-slip floor mats beside beds at night, and turn on night lights to illuminate the path between the bed and bathroom. Nurses observing individuals in restraint can suggest safety improvements for surrounding areas.

Be knowledgeable about the organization's equipment preventive maintenance programs and double check to help ensure equipment safety. All direct care nursing staff should be knowledgeable about existing equipment preventive maintenance programs. By examining restraint equipment and appropriate documents for the performance of routine and preventive maintenance, nursing staff can serve as an additional check point to ensure that preventive maintenance has been completed as required. When nurses find cases where equipment has not been maintained as required, they should be knowledgeable about who to notify and how. Similarly, if nurses observe equipment that needs repair, they should know where to go to get a replacement, how to remove the defective equipment from use, and how to notify maintenance per-

sonnel to pick up the equipment and make repairs. Home health staff, therapists, aides and companions can also be educated about this process. Nurses in the home care setting can help ensure that information about the equipment and how to reach its vendor is placed in the home care recipient's chart.

Root Cause 3: Inadequate Observation/ Monitoring Procedures or Practices

Sentinel Event Example: Inadequate Monitoring.

A man receiving care in a behavioral health care facility experiences severe delirium, tremors, and hallucinations and begins to exhibit difficult and dangerous behavior. While arranging to transfer the man to an appropriate acute care setting, staff are concerned about his safety and the safety of those around him. They try a variety of alternatives to the use of restraint but each alternative is unsuccessful. The staff place the man in 4-point restraint in the only area not currently occupied—a private room far from the nursing station. Since staffing is in short supply that evening, no staff member is available to remain with the man. The charge nurse intends to return every five minutes for observations. However, other critical situations develop and the nurse does not return for almost one hour. At that time, the nurse finds the man unresponsive, having suffered a heart attack. He also has huge welts on all four extremities.

In order to prevent injury, individuals in restraints must be adequately monitored. If a restraint is used for too long, and if the individual is unable to move, health problems can occur, including pressure ulcers, nerve damage, and incontinence.[4] Psychological and physical decline can also occur as illustrated in the example above. Continuous observation of individuals in restraint can effectively reduce restraint-related deaths and injuries. Properly trained ancillary or volunteer staff, such as sitters, can be used to provide this one-on-one observation.

Organization leaders must ensure thorough monitoring policies and procedures, including proper documentation of observation. Policies and procedures should address how frequently individuals in restraints should be observed. Requirements vary from program to program;

one organization policy may not serve the needs of all programs. Organizations must be certain that their policies provide enough detail regarding observation procedures. All nursing staff working in organizations with multiple programs and providing care in multiple settings should be competent with all policies and procedures.

Prevention Strategies

Observe individuals receiving care. One of the most effective methods of preventing the need for restraint is increased observation and supervision of care recipients by nursing staff. For example, frequent monitoring of cognitively impaired individuals can alert staff members to early signs of restlessness or agitation. This may signal an increase in pain or discomfort which can be addressed before restraints or alternatives are necessary. High-risk individuals can be located close to nurses' areas to allow regular observation.

Nurses can identify individuals who are incontinent or who have the need to urinate frequently and place them on a prompted voiding schedule that allows for them to empty their bladder at least every two hours. A staff member will need to remind the individual to go to the bathroom and possibly even assist them with the toileting. This should be done even if the individual does not feel the urge to void at that time. Scheduled toileting reduces anxiety about the need to void and can decrease wandering by individuals looking for the bathroom because they feel their bladder is full but are not able to express their needs well.

Consistently observe individuals in restraint, according to organization policies and procedures. Nursing staff should be vigilant about observing individuals in restraint and documenting their observations according to the policies and procedures established by the organization. Many organizations train staff to evaluate through observation not only whether the individual is safe, but whether the individual can be taken out of restraint. One behavioral health care organization that provides services to children and adolescents trained staff members to ask themselves the "COPING" questions:[6]

- Is the individual in **C**ontrol?
- Is the staff member and individual **O**riented to the circumstances around restraint use?
- Can the staff member and individual identify a **P**attern as to why and when the circumstances occurred?
- Having made a connection with the individual, can alternatives be **I**nvestigated?
- Will the individual **N**egotiate, or do things differently so that this won't happen again?
- Can the staff member **G**ive control back to the individual?

Control is given back to the individual through teaching alternative skills to those that made restraint necessary. Continuous observation of individuals in restraint significantly reduces the likelihood of adverse events.

Root Cause 4: Inadequate Assessment/ Reassessment

Sentinel Event Example: Incomplete Assessment.

An organization delivering care for post surgical sub-acute patients admits a small, elderly gentleman at 2:00 PM. The man had a hip replaced three days earlier and still shows signs of confusion. The day shift nurse, with less than one hour remaining to work, performs the admission nursing assessment. She notes on the admitting physician's orders that the man is still slightly confused. The attending physician orders a waist restraint and the placement of bedrails in the raised position while the man is in bed. The physician is concerned that the man will attempt to walk and bear full weight on the operative hip too soon and possibly cause damage to the new hip prosthesis.

Shortly before 3:00 PM, the nurse applies the waist restraint, raises the bedrails, and leaves to give report to the next shift. She fails to indicate in her assessment an increased safety danger due to differences in the type of beds and bedrails used on this unit and the small physical size of the elderly gentleman.

After receiving report, the nurse on the 3:00 PM to 11:00 PM shift immediately checks the man. She finds him without vital signs, cold, blue and with his head and neck caught in the larger size bedrails. Efforts to perform CPR on the man are futile. Less than two hours after admission, he is dead from asphyxiation.

The initial assessment process determines what kind of care is required to meet an individual's initial needs. The reassessment process evaluates the individual's continuing needs that change in response to care and treatment. Timely and accurate completion of assessments and reassessments by all caregiving disciplines can identify opportunities to improve the individual's overall status, thereby eliminating or reducing the need for restraint. Accurate assessment allows a proactive evaluation of possible alternatives to restraint should it be indicated during treatment. Failure to complete assessments within the time frames specified by organization policies and procedures is a continuing problem in many health care organizations. Without proper and timely assessment, care planning and provision cannot be on target.

Prevention Strategies

Identify and remove contraband. On admission, nursing staff can help ensure that any and all contraband items, such as matches and other smoking materials, drugs, alcohol, and sharp objects, are removed from care recipient access and access by family and friends. Nurses should also monitor material brought in by visitors.

Assess and reassess all individuals in a timely and thorough manner, according to organization policies and procedures. To reduce the risk of restraint-related injury or death, nursing assessments must be performed in a timely manner for new admissions. In addition, nursing reassessments documenting changes in care recipient conditions while in restraint must be performed and documented in a timely manner. The age and gender of care recipients—highly correlated with increased risk of restraint-related death or injury—must be considered. A description of specific assessment needs follows. Any and all adverse or "unusual" effects of medications should be noted in the clinical record.

Adequately assess care recipient's nutritional status. Nutritional status can directly affect an individual's level of cognition which, in turn, can directly affect the need for restraint. Timely identification and treatment of nutritional issues such as dehydration and malnutrition by nursing and dietitian staff can improve the cognitive status of care recipients. Particularly with the elderly, timely assessment and treatment of nutritional status can decrease or eliminate the need to use restraint.[7]

Adequately assess pain management needs of the care recipient. Many attempts to get out of restraints and resulting injuries and deaths are motivated by the care recipient's need for maximum comfort and relief of pain.[8] Some individuals with cognitive impairments may exhibit agitated or aggressive behavior when experiencing pain. Nurses should assess pain on admission and reassess on an ongoing basis.

Accurately assess care recipient's toileting needs. Attempts to get out of restraints often are also motivated by the individual's need to eliminate urine or stool. Nurses should assess the care recipient's bowel and bladder functions and develop a care plan that meets toileting needs.

Help to ensure accurate assessment of the care recipient's mental cognition. The nursing assessment should identify individuals with cognitive issues. Inadequate perception of surroundings, mental disorientation, and other cognitive issues can lead to the use of restraint. These care recipients may need to be evaluated by professionals in other disciplines. Putting a restraint on certain individuals with cognitive impairment can heighten their care needs, not reduce them. For example, a chronically agitated individual might become more agitated when physically restrained. Care plans that include restraint alternatives can be developed and implemented by nursing staff.

Accurately assess the care recipient's physical strength. Through timely assessment and care planning, nurses can help to ensure that physically weak individuals participate in muscle-strengthening programs to improve sitting balance and eliminate the need for restraint.

Identify restraint alternatives. Educate family members. Through the assessment process, nurses can assist in identifying care recipients who may do well with measures other than physical restraints (see Sidebar 6-3, page 75, mentioned earlier in this chapter). An in-depth nursing assessment and family interview provide the necessary background information. Education of family members can facilitate family cooperation in providing one-on-one supervision so that physical restraints do not need to be used. Family members can be taught therapeutic holding techniques that help to reduce the need for restraint or seclusion.

Accurately assess each individual for the appropriateness of restraint use. Nursing assessments must be customized for each individual. If an individual requires restraint, nursing staff should identify the cause of the need for restraint and relate this to other assessment factors before communicating the need for restraint. For example, in acute care, where restraints are most often used to prevent falls or to maintain therapy, nurses can evaluate care recipients who refuse to stay in bed for cognitive status, performance of activities of daily living, agitation, the presence of psychotropic drugs, and incidence of falls.[9] Restraint alternatives should be considered.

Root Cause 5: Inadequate Care Planning or Provision

"Near Miss" Example: Inadequate Provision of Care. *A woman is hospitalized in the intensive care unit following a motor vehicle accident. With multiple broken bones and closed head trauma, she requires multiple IV lines, a foley catheter, a cardiac monitor, and artificial ventilation. She also experienced severe seizures while being treated in the emergency room. The woman's medical orders include an order for both hands to be restrained at all times.*

On day two of caring for this individual, the nurse notes that the woman has had no further seizures and currently, is lying calmly in the bed. After completing several tasks at the bedside, the nurse needs to dispose of some equipment away from the bedside, but still in the room. In an effort to save time, the nurse places both side rails in the raised position but does not restrain the woman's upper extremities. With her back to the woman and on the opposite side of the room, the nurse hears slight movement. Returning quickly to the bedside, she discovers that in a brief amount of time, the woman has pulled out her foley catheter with one hand and dislodged the IV lines with the other hand. The nurse is able to correct the situation promptly.

Organization leaders must ensure that care, treatment, and rehabilitation are planned and appropriate to the individual's needs. Then,

health care staff must provide the care and treatment, as planned. Effective care and treatment reduces the likelihood of restraint use and concomitant risk of death and injury. Communication to all caregivers of the care plan goals and the approaches to those goals must be effective. Involvement and education of the individual and family about goals and approaches help to reduce the likelihood of adverse events.

Prevention Strategies

Ensure appropriate time limits for restraint orders. Nurses can help ensure compliance with requirements related to time limits for restraint orders and the organization's policy and process for face-to-face evaluation by licensed independent practitioners.

Ensure proper use of physical restraint techniques. Nurses should be knowledgeable about proper restraint techniques and help to ensure that all caregiving staff use such techniques. For example, experts recommend the following:

- If an individual is restrained in the supine position (lying face upwards), ensure that the head is free to rotate to the side, and when possible, the head of the bed is elevated to minimize the risk of aspiration.

- If an individual is restrained in the prone position (lying face downwards), ensure that the airway is unobstructed at all times. For example, do not cover or "bury" the individual's face. Also ensure that expansion of the individual's lungs is not restricted by excessive pressure on the individual's back. Special caution is required for children, elderly individuals, and obese individuals.

- Never place a towel, bag, or other cover over an individual's face as part of the therapeutic holding process.

- Do not restrain an individual in a bed with unprotected split side rails.

- Discontinue use of certain types of restraints, such as high vests and waist restraints.

Nursing staff also need to be aware of the danger of using restraints and holds with individuals with severe osteoporosis. Use of many types of restraints and therapeutic holding are contraindicated with such individuals due to the fragility of their bones.

Concluding Comments

Using physical restraints is dangerous. Nurses can reduce the likelihood of restraint-related deaths or injuries by using alternatives to restraint, whenever possible, ensuring proper training and competence assessment, accurately assessing and reassessing individuals in restraint, using restraint equipment safely, and thoroughly monitoring individuals in restraint.

References

1. Joint Commission: *Reducing Restraint Use in the Acute Care Environment.* Oakbrook Terrace, IL: Joint Commission on Accreditation of Healthcare Organizations, 1998, p. iv.

2. Joint Commission: *Lexikon: Dictionary of Health Care Terms, Organizations, and Acronyms, 2nd Edition.* Oakbrook Terrace, IL: Joint Commission on Accreditation of Healthcare Organizations, 1998.

3. Food and Drug Administration: Safe use of physical restraint devices. *FDA Backgrounder,* Jul 1992.

4. Weiss EM: A nationwide pattern of death. *The Hartford Courant,* Oct 11, 1998.

5. Joint Commission: Preventing restraint deaths. *Sentinel Event Alert* Issue 8, Nov 18, 1998.

6. Joint Commission: *Preventing Adverse Events in Behavioral Health Care: A Systems Approach to Sentinel Events.* Oakbrook Terrace, IL: Joint Commission on Accreditation of Healthcare Organizations, 1999, p 106.

7. Gainey A: Caregiving: Focus on reducing restraints in SNFs. *Provider* 26(7):49–50, 2000.

8. Howard-Ruben J: A new respect for pain. *Nursing Spectrum* 13(14):12–13, 2000.

9. Werner P, et al: Individualized care alternatives used in the process of removing physical restraints in the nursing home. *J Am Geriatr Soc* 42:321–325, 1994.

Chapter 7:

Preventing Serious Injury or Death Following Elopement

The death or serious injury of an individual who has eloped from a health care facility presents double jeopardy for organizations. Not only has the individual managed to leave the facility without permission, but once beyond the facility's walls, the individual was seriously injured or died. *Elopement* is defined as the departure of an individual, without permission, from the physical boundaries of a health care organization.[1] Other terms for elopement include "absent without leave" (AWOL) and "away without authorization" (AWA).

Cause for Concern

When an individual who is compromised by psychiatric or organic illness elopes from a health care setting, his or her treatment is interrupted, increasing the likelihood of negative care outcomes as well as the risk of a sentinel event. Behavioral health care settings are familiar with this issue. Studies published in the professional literature indicate that 3% to 15% of individuals admitted to psychiatric facilities elope each year.[2] Facilities that treat the elderly and the developmentally disabled are also familiar with this problem. Individuals with cognitive impairment resulting from Alzheimer's, dementia, and developmental disabilities are at high risk for elopement.

Thankfully, not all elopements result in sentinel events. However, serious injuries and deaths following elopement happen with significant frequency. In fact, death following elopement is the ninth most frequently indicated type of sentinel event reviewed by the

Joint Commission, accounting for approximately 3% of sentinel events reviewed.

The key to preventing serious injuries and deaths following elopement is to prevent elopement. Individuals elope for a variety of reasons, frequently related to one or more problems in the individual's cognitive, emotional, social, or physical condition. Preventing elopement and resulting serious injuries or deaths requires on-target interdisciplinary assessment, planning, and care provision. Nurses play a key role in these processes. As managers and caregivers in 24-hour care settings, nurses provide care to individuals day-in and day-out. They are able to note changes in mental or physical status that could potentially lead to an elopement. They are keenly aware of environmental or staffing issues that can increase the incidence of elopement. As front-line providers, they most frequently are responsible for implementing elopement prevention plans.

Root Causes and Prevention Strategies

Environment of care issues, inadequate assessment, insufficient staff training, and inadequate communication are frequently cited as root causes for deaths and serious injuries following elopement. A thorough look at each root cause and prevention strategies nurses can use follows. Sidebar 7-1, page 84, provides additional strategies recommended by the Centers for Medicare and Medicaid (CMS) (formerly HCFA) to prevent elopement from continuing care facilities. Most of these can be implemented by nurses in all health care settings.

SIDEBAR 7-1. PREVENTING ELOPEMENT: CMS RECOMMENDATIONS

- Establish protocols to identify potential wanderers upon admission to nursing, rehabilitation, or other continuing care facilities.

- Continue wandering assessment into the first few days of the resident's stay— remember that elopement attempts are most likely to occur in the first two to three days.

- Carefully document in the resident's chart all admission information received from the resident's family or from other institutions, and the results of independent assessments or observations with respect to wandering, confusion, or elopement attempts.

- Document notes on safety precautions taken at the time (for example, additional supervision, room placement, electronic triggering devices, restraints).

- Make sure all caregivers are aware of an individual's propensity to wander. Ensure communication of wandering or elopement attempts from one nursing shift to the next.

- Implement the wandering prevention and management strategies appropriate for the facility.

- If electronic devices and alarms are used, ensure that staff are trained in their use, and investigate each time they are activated.

- Consult local fire safety regulations before installing any automatic locking device on exit or other doors.

- Have a protocol in place to locate missing patients or residents. Ensure that all staff are familiar with the procedure. Conduct drills regularly.

- Review restraint and seclusion policies for violent or psychotic patients in all facilities. Ensure that these patients are closely supervised.

- Ensure that adequate documentation is completed.

Source: Health Care Financing Administration: Additional Guidance to Surveyors *Life Safety Code.* Memorandum. Mar 10, 1994.

Root Cause 1: Unsafe Environment of Care

Sentinel Event Example: Unattended Exits. *An adult general psychiatry inpatient unit begins to admit adolescents with acute psychiatric symptoms. Exit doors on the unit are locked. The locks open automatically when the fire alarm is activated. This has never posed a safety issue in the past. A 16-year old adolescent girl with major depression, suicide ideation, and a history of substance abuse is admitted to the unit. On the night shift, this girl pulls the fire alarm and leaves through an exit door. By the time the staff realizes that she is missing, the girl is off the facility's grounds. Her body is found several days later in a nearby river. She apparently died after jumping from a bridge.*

Sentinel Event Example: Unmonitored Exits. *In a large long term care unit for individuals with dementia, the exits are equipped with cameras that can be monitored from the nursing station. The unit doors are locked and there is a bell on the outside for visitors to request access to the unit. A group of visitors arrives and the nursing staff buzzes them in. The nurse at the nursing station is quite busy and does not continuously observe the monitor while the visitors are entering the unit. While the door is held open for the visitors, a well dressed resident with dementia exits the unit. He dies after being struck by a car while crossing a highway near the facility.*

Problems with the safety of the physical environment of care are frequently implicated in elopements. The fact that the care recipient is able to leave the facility indicates that security measures failed. As consistent with high-quality health care, organizations are now placing a greater emphasis on the least restrictive level of care. Although appropriate, this emphasis, when combined with the increased acuity of individuals in their care, can lead to higher elopement risk. The first example above illustrates what could happen when an organization does not make adjustments to its security plan as care recipient needs change. The second example illustrates how staff must be vigilant in their use of security systems.

To determine appropriate security measures, the organization needs to conduct risk assessment activities. In planning for and providing security measures, leaders and organization staff must consider the individual's rights, including privacy, and the need for a therapeutic environment. On units that treat individuals with dementia, basic measures, such as a brightly colored band across an exit or elevators, may be sufficient to prevent individuals from wandering. Other care settings might need a higher level of environmental control, such as that afforded by electronic movement systems. Individuals in organizations using these systems wear an electronic band or tag that contains a sensor that locks the exit doors or sounds an alarm if the individual approaches a door.[3] Psychiatric units typically use locked doors and may also use cameras to monitor movement. Staff must select the most effective system for *that* organization's population, as identified through the risk assessment process.

Prevention Strategies

Know and apply the organization's safety and security measures. As providers of much of the direct care given to individuals in health care facilities, nurses can have a major impact on the prevention of death and serious injury following elopement as a result of elopement. Nursing staff need to be well versed in the safety and security measures in their work environment and help ensure that those measures are applied consistently.

Report unsafe aspects of the care environment. Nurses have a good sense about how the environment supports or jeopardizes care safety. They provide feedback to organization leaders and the staff responsible for environmental services regarding safety incidents that occur. By reporting safety equipment malfunctions, improvement needs, and all safety incidents, whether or not resulting in an injury or other

adverse occurrence, nurses help the organization to monitor the effectiveness of its safety and security measures. For example, nurses should report all incidents of an individual eloping from the unit, even though that person returns to the unit unharmed.

Root Cause 2: Inadequate Assessment

Sentinel Event Example: Inadequate Initial Assessment. *A 40-year-old man is admitted to a psychiatric unit after physically attacking another resident at the homeless shelter where he was spending the night. The shelter staff indicated that they had felt threatened by the man's behavior for several days. The man has a psychiatric history, but this is his first admission to the unit, and no history is available to unit staff. The man is very guarded about providing information, prefers to be alone, and communicates very little to others on the unit. During his first hours on the unit, he exhibits no aggressive behavior. Staff members do not initiate special observation procedures because during the assessment process, the man denies suicide and homicide ideation. Two days after admission, the man receives privileges to leave the unit to smoke. He then escapes the facility while out on a cigarette break, and returns to the homeless shelter where he murders the resident that he had previously attacked prior to admission. He then kills himself.*

Sentinel Event Example: Inadequate Reassessment. *Nursing staff in a long term care facility note that an 80-year old woman with a history of progressive dementia is unusually irritable and restless. She is pacing, talking in a loud voice, and complaining about a number of issues. The nurses on duty are unable to appease her or to determine the cause of what they view as a "bad mood." Staff members frequently remind the woman to move away from the exit door. In the evening, the staff discover that the woman is no longer on the unit, nor in the building. The woman left the facility without warm clothing on a cold evening with sub zero temperatures. She is found dead the following morning in a wooded area near the facility. Her death was caused by exposure.*

Both examples illustrate how inadequate assessment and reassessment can lead to death following elopement. By relying solely on information provided by the care recipient, staff in the first example did not accurately assess the individual's at-risk-for-elopement status and need for special observation procedures. Similarly, staff in the second example did not reassess the woman's care needs and therefore missed the fact that she was at increased risk for elopement.

Thorough initial assessment procedures must be in place to identify the risk of elopement.[2] The literature emphasizes the importance of being able to identify elopement risk factors, predictive behavior, and development and implementation of appropriate interventions to prevent elopement. A complete history and assessment of the individual's current functioning, mental status, and desire for treatment are important in identifying factors that may lead to elopement. Reports and studies appearing in the literature have identified characteristics and treatment factors associated with elopement. For example, one study[4] indicates that young males or females with a persistent mental illness who have a history of psychotic, impulsive behavior are at the highest risk for elopement from a psychiatric unit. Also at risk are individuals with a family history of abusive, violent behavior. Other authors site a correlation between involuntary hospitalization and elopement.[5]

Prevention Strategies

Ensure the thorough initial assessment of each individual for elopement risk. A comprehensive initial assessment by qualified professionals, including nurses, can identify problems that could lead to elopement due to a care recipient's behavioral disorder, fear, poor judgment, or lack of insight. Problems in these areas will place the individual at great risk for harm if he or she leaves the facility's protective environment. Nurses can improve their ability to identify individuals at risk for elopement by being familiar with current elopement studies and literature. Nurses also can identify factors unique to the organization's population that could characterize an individual at risk for elopement. For example, individuals with dementia have a high risk of elopement due to confusion, disorientation, and at times, agitation. Nurses can use this knowledge to ensure the development and implementation of program and care plans that address symptoms and behaviors that occur with dementia, thereby minimizing elopement risk.

Ensure regular reassessment of each individual for elopement risk. Reassessment identifies an individual's response to care. Nurses have the opportunity to observe the individual and note any changes in condition that might increase the risk of elopement. Changes in mental status can be a predictor of dangerous behavior such as elopement. Staff assignments need to reflect an increased need for observation that might be indicated for an individual who is at high risk for elopement. Nursing staff in some facilities have used current knowledge and internal quality improvement data to develop observation documentation forms (checklists) that staff use to determine risk factors for elopement.[5] These checklists are completed daily or more frequently to assess care recipients. Aggregated data from the checklists can be used to monitor issues involved in an elopement. Family members need to be informed of the risk for elopement to assure that they will follow good safety practices when visiting. Nurses can enlist the family's help in developing and providing an individualized safety plan.

Continuous reassessment is critical. A change in the individual's mental status or treatment, or a change in staffing patterns could lead to an increased potential for elopement.[6] Ongoing observation and assessment are also important because individuals may not be willing or able to provide information during the initial assessment. Intensive observation through increased checks or one-to-one monitoring carried out by the nursing staff provides a basic intervention technique used by many organizations. The behavioral checklist used by one organization to document observations appears as Figure 7-1, page 87.

Help to ensure the proper linkage of assessment data and care planning/provision. Care planning must be responsive to the specific care that an individual needs. Nursing staff can help to ensure that assessment data are integrated in the care planning and provision processes. For example, if an individual with dementia is admitted to a long term care organization, nursing staff must plan for the provision of orienting devices at exits, such as a stop sign, or a brightly colored band across the elevators to manage wandering. Activities and structure on the unit will keep

Behavioral Checklist

Veterans Administration

Ward: 1A   **Date:** 11/9/90

Patient Names	6A	7A	8A	9A	10A	11A	12P	1P	2P	3P	4P	5P	6P	7P	8P	9P	10P
A	26	11 / 21	20	25	23	24	20	28	14	7 / 19	19	20	11 / 26	26	26	26	26
B	26	1.2 / 10	20	1.2 / 27.8	21 / 8	14 / 19	20	11 / 26	26	26	26	11 / 20	11 / 27	11 / 27	14 / 19	26	26
C	26 / 18	5.6 / 18	21 / 18	21.18 / 27	21 / 28	21 / 18	21 / 20	9.19	21 / 16	11 / 17	26	26	21 / 20	11 / 27	11 / 27	26	26
D	11 / 27	11 / 27	24	24	23	28	24	21 / 27	27	24	27	27	24	11 / 27	11 / 27	11 / 27	26
E	14 / 27	14 / 27	19 / 27	26	26	11 / 27	24	24	23	11 / 27	11 / 27	24	24	11 / 27	11 / 27	11 / 27	26
F	22 / 27	22 / 27	20 / 27	22 / 23	28	22 / 27	20 / 27	26	26	22 / 27	22 / 27	22 / 27	22 / 27	22 / 27	22 / 27	22 / 27	26
G	26	11 / 27	24	28	23	24	24	11 / 27	11 / 27	11 / 27	11 / 27	24	24	21 / 27	27	27	26
H	1.2 / 27	1.2 / 27	21 / 20	1.2 / 27	1.2 / 27	1.2 / 27	21 / 27	20 / 27	26	26	26	1.2 / 27	1.2 / 27	1.2 / 27	21 / 27	26	26

Care and Observation Code:

1. Confused	11. Quiet	21. No Change in Mental Status
2. Disoriented	12. Cursing	22. Withdrawn/Seclusive
3. Delusional	13. Combative	23. Group Therapy
4. Hallucinating	14. Pacing/Restless	24. Off Ward
5. Hostile	15. Standing Still/Catatonic	25. Clinic Appointment
6. Threatening	16. Placed in Seclusion	26. Asleep
7. Suspicious	17. Out of Seclusion	27. In Dayroom
8. Fluids Offered	18. 1:1 Observation	28. With Physician
9. Yelling/Screaming	19. PRN Meds Given	29. Talking with staff/peers
10. Mumbling Incoherently	20. Meal Served	30.

Figure 7-1. *Sample of a Behavioral Checklist.* **Source:** *Richmond I, Dandridge L, Jones K: Changing nursing practice to prevent elopement.* Journal of Nursing Care Quality *6(1):73–81, 1991. Used with permission.*

individuals engaged therapeutically, will help manage anxiety, and will facilitate observation of several persons at the same time.

Root Cause 3: Inadequate Staff Orientation and Training

Sentinel Event Example: Inadequate Orientation. *A man restricted to the psychiatric unit of an acute care organization asks an agency nurse hired to work one shift if he can join the group leaving the unit for a cigarette break. It is the nurse's first day on the unit, and he has not yet received an orientation to the facility. Specific orientation materials are not provided to agency staff, but the nurse received a brief orientation from a nurse manager permanently assigned to the unit. The agency nurse does not recall hearing that the man is at risk for elopement, and as such, is placed "on level one." Not familiar with the level system, the nurse does not realize that this means that the man is confined to the unit. He takes the man and four others for a cigarette break. The man flees the group during the break, leaves the facility, and is found dead later that day in the garage of his home, a victim of carbon monoxide poisoning.*

Unfamiliar with basic safety precautions, such as observation protocols, privilege levels, and providing an assessment specific to the organization's population, untrained staff represent a risk to safety and increase the likelihood of sentinel events related to elopement. A well-educated staff is better prepared to predict and prevent elopements. All staff, including agency and per diem staff, need to be oriented to the policies and procedures in their departments and in the organization. Nursing staff need to be competent in assessing care recipients for elopement risk and developing and implementing treatment plans that address the risk of elopement. Nursing staff also need to be educated about the security and safety measures in the environment of care. For example, if electronic devices and alarms are used, nurses must be trained in their application and maintenance needs.

Prevention Strategies

Know elopement risk factors and who is at risk for elopement. As mentioned previously, the literature is full of research and studies about predicting and preventing elopement. Nursing staff need to be well educated about current

research and practices found to minimize elopement risk. They also need to be well informed of individuals in their care who are at risk for elopement.

Ensure competence in implementing the organization's assessment, planning, and care provision for individuals at risk for elopement. Nurses must feel comfortable about their personal competence to assess and care for individuals at risk for elopement. If uncomfortable with their competence level, nurses should request additional training. If units use screening tools or special protocols or checklists (see Figure 7-1, page 87) to respond to individuals who are at risk for elopement, staff must be trained in their use. All staff who work in the area need to be oriented to any special documentation or procedures to assure the safety of individuals on particular units. In order to promote safety, nursing staff need to be aware of specific unit or organizationwide safety policies, procedures, and devices.

Maintain ongoing competence in assessing and caring for individuals at risk for elopement. Nurses must ensure that they maintain current skills and obtain new skills to reflect the changing needs of individuals in their care and current best practices. Leaders must ensure that specific competencies for nursing staff are identified and evaluated on a regular basis. Education should be provided to prepare staff to deal with populations new to the organization. Many behavioral health care and other facilities and units are treating individuals who have more acute symptoms and are more disabled, but whose lengths of stay are shorter. Nurses need to develop new skills to effectively treat these individuals. Working with more disabled care recipients, for example, nurses may encounter more problems with treatment noncompliance, escapes, aggression, and self-destructive behavior. Regular in-services and competence assessment will help ensure that the nursing staff has the skills necessary to predict and adequately plan to prevent sentinel events following elopement.

Root Cause 4: Inadequate Communication

Sentinel Event Example: Inadequate Communication Between Staff and Patient. *A 50-year old male is admitted to a behavioral health care facility with acute symptoms of depression, suicide* *ideation, and substance abuse. He reports that his wife recently left him due to her frustration regarding his long history of substance abuse and depression. While in the facility, the man receives a call from his wife informing him that she is filing for divorce. In an individual session with a counselor, the man reports his conversation with his wife. He is quite agitated, depressed, and tearful, and expresses homicidal ideation towards his wife. The counselor believes the man is just expressing his shock at the loss of his marriage. The counselor plans to write a detailed note about the session at the end of the shift. He does not verbally report the conversation to any other staff members. It is a very busy evening and staff do not have the opportunity to meet. Later that evening, the depressed man is found to be missing from the unit. Several hours later, the police arrive to question unit staff. They inform the staff that the man murdered his wife and then killed himself.*

Multidisciplinary communication is key to reducing the likelihood of elopement and resulting deaths or injuries. Poor communication, such as that illustrated in the previous example can lead to sentinel events. All staff must have critical information about care recipients at risk for elopement and changes in condition that might indicate increased risk. Staff communication that ensures the availability of all appropriate information must be ongoing and thorough.

Prevention Strategies

Communicate and document critical information about at risk individuals. Preventing elopement requires the combined efforts of a multidisciplinary staff. As key team members and caregivers, nurses must communicate to other caregivers information regarding individuals at risk for elopement. Documentation in the clinical record is essential, but verbal communication facilitates information transfer. Since elopement can be precipitated by problems in any area of functioning, staff with expertise and responsibilities for particular areas of the care plan need to work together to provide the safest and most therapeutic plan. This involves extensive verbal and written communication. Staff on all shifts must be informed of specific plans. Some units have methods, such as specially colored identification bands, to identify those at risk for elopement. Nursing staff can communicate special

safety plans through the nursing report, which all staff should be required to hear prior to beginning work. The report can be taped if necessary to assure the information's availability to all staff. Communication following an elopement is also vital. One behavioral health unit described in the professional literature uses a questionnaire to facilitate the transfer of critical information following an elopement. This appears as Figure 7-2, page 90.

Participate in team meetings. Nursing presence and communication at team meetings is essential. Nurses must share their observations and assessments of individuals, and add their expertise to the development of a workable and individualized safety plan for each care recipient. In the ideal world, all staff providing care to individuals at risk for elopement should participate in team meetings. At times, this may not be possible due to the need to provide coverage on the unit. Nurses can help ensure that all front line staff, such as nurses aides and counselors, who spend considerable time providing direct care, receive information vital to the continued safety of individuals in their care. For example, such staff should receive information regarding signs and symptoms to look for, and details of the treatment plan. If an individual's condition changes and there is a new risk of elopement, nurses should update team members using the communication methods established by the organization. Staff in some organizations participate in brief daily rounds as an updating mechanism. A special team meeting can be considered if a new risk is identified, so that the multidisciplinary staff can revise the treatment plan.

Concluding Comments

Individuals who are unable to care for themselves due to organic illnesses, dementia, or psychiatric problems are at risk for harm when they escape from the protection offered by a health care organization. Health care leaders and staff have a responsibility to protect individuals at risk of harm due to elopement. Assessment, planning, observation, and care provided by the nursing staff are critical to preventing sentinel events following elopement.

Sample Elopement Questionnaire

Date_____   Ward_____

Instructions: This questionnaire is to be completed by the charge nurse immediately after an elopement occurs. Please deposit the completed questionnaires in the envelope labeled "Elopements."

1. Diagnosis _____

2. Mental status when elopement occurred. Check any of the following that were applicable:

   A. Suicidal ideation   E. Hallucinations
   B. Homicidal ideation   F. Disorientation
   C. Threatening behavior toward other people   G. Delusional thinking
   D. Confusion   H. Hostile/suspicious

3. Does this patient have a history of previous elopements? Yes____ No____

4. Were there any verbal indications given by the patient that he may be planning to elope? Yes____ No____
   If yes, please describe. Include statements such as "needing to be at home, or feeling that hospitalization is not needed." _____
   _____
   _____

5. Were there any nonverbal clues given by the patient such as constantly standing by or watching the door? Yes____ No____ If yes, please describe._____
   _____
   _____

6. What was the ward census at the time of the elopement? _____

7. What time did the elopement occur? _____

8. Was the door locked or unlocked when the elopement occurred? _____

9. Were nursing staff present at the door when the elopement occurred? Yes____ No____

10. Was this patient a voluntary admission or was he committed? _____

11. Was the ward unusually busy at the time of the elopement, such as show of force in progress or a medical emergency? Yes____ No____

12. Did the patient have off-ward privileges? Yes____ No____

13. If the patient had privileges, did he elope while off the ward on privileges? Yes____ No____

Figure 7-2. Sample elopement questionnaire. ***Source:*** *Richmond I, Dandridge L, Jones K: Changing nursing practice to prevent elopement.* Journal of Nursing Care Quality *6(1):73–81, 1991. Used with permission.*

References

1. McIndoe KI: Elope: Why psychiatric patients go AWOL. *Journal of Psychosocial Nursing* 26:16–20, 1986.

2. Platts WE: Psychiatric patients: Premises liability and predicting patient elopement. *Journal of Healthcare Protection Management* 14(2):66–77, 1998.

3. Bowers DM: Closing the door on wanderers. *Journal of Healthcare Protection Management* 15(1): 109–117, 1998/1999.

4. Smith TE, Munich RL: Suicide, violence, and elopement: Prediction, understanding, and management. *Hospital Psychiatry* 11:534–535; 1992.

5. Richmond I, Dandridge L, Jones K: Changing nursing practice to prevent elopement. *Journal of Nursing Care Quality* 6(1):73–81, 1991.

6. Kashubeck S, et al: Predicting elopement from residential treatment centers. *American Journal of Orthopsychiatry* 64(1):126–135, 1994.

Chapter 8:

Preventing Suicide

Inpatient suicide. These words strike terror in the hearts of health care professionals nationwide. Hospitals and other 24-hour facilities are places for quality treatment and care. They are meant to be safe. How could suicide occur in such settings?

Cause for Concern

Every 17.1 minutes, one American commits suicide. Now the eighth leading cause of death in the United States, more than 31,000 people take their lives each year. Another approximately 775,000 people attempt it, resulting in an estimated 5 million suicide survivors in the United States.[1] Approximately 2% to 6% of suicides are by individuals receiving treatment from health care professionals in a hospital setting.[2] Suicidal behaviors are far more common among individuals receiving health care services than in the population at large. Approximately 12 persons per 100,000 commit suicide in the general population; in hospital settings, the rates range from 40 to 350 per 100,000 inpatients.[3] Studies indicate that of those persons committing a suicide, 50% saw a physician in the weeks prior to completing the act.[4]

Suicidality is the most common reason for psychiatric inpatient admission. Reports indicate that between 60% and 75% of child, adolescent, and adult care recipients and 40% to 55% of geriatric care recipients are admitted to inpatient units with concerns of self-harm.[5] A considerable amount of research exists on the occurrence of suicide in hospital settings. Norman Farberow[3] and Robert Litman[6] found that approximately one-third of inpatients who commit suicide do so while on an authorized pass from a health care facility, another third

after eloping from the unit, and the final third while within the unit itself. On units, the most frequent suicide method is hanging; the next most frequent is jumping from a window or rooftop. Firearms are the most common method used outside the unit. Bathrooms are the most common site of inpatient suicide, followed by the individual's room.[3,7,8] High-risk periods occur during times of transition for the individual, including shortly after admission and just prior to or following discharge.[6,7]

Since implementation of the Sentinel Event Policy in 1995, suicide is the number one type of sentinel event reviewed by the Joint Commission. Of the nearly 1,100 sentinel events reviewed from 1995 through early 2001, nearly 200 (18%) were inpatient suicides. Most of these suicides occurred in psychiatric hospitals and psychiatric units of general hospitals and to a lesser degree in medical/surgical units of acute general hospitals.[9] Some occurred in residential care facilities. In the vast majority of these cases, the method of suicide chosen by the individual was hanging in a bathroom, bedroom, or closet. In about 20% of the cases, individuals jumped to their death from a roof or out of a window. Organizations that experienced inpatient suicides reviewed by the Joint Commission identified the following issues as root causes:

- Patient assessment methods, such as incomplete suicide risk assessment at intake, absent or incomplete reassessment, and incomplete examination of the individual (for example, failure to identify a contraband).

- The environment of care, such as the presence of non-breakaway bars, rods or safety rails; lack of testing of breakaway hardware; and inadequate security.

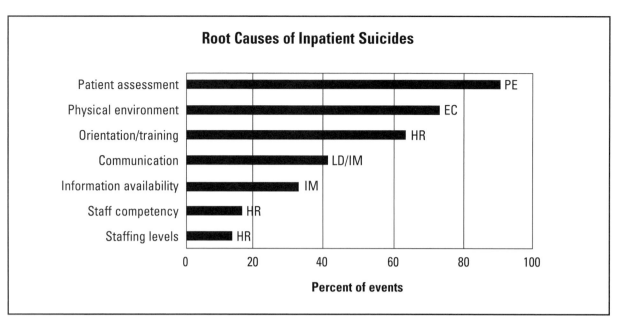

Figure 8-1. *This chart illustrates the percentage of causes at the root of suicides reported to the Joint Commission between January 1995 and January 2001.*

- Staff-related factors, such as insufficient orientation or training, incomplete competency review or credentialing, and inadequate staffing levels.

- Information-related factors such as incomplete communication among caregivers and information being unavailable when needed.

- Care planning, such as assignment of the care recipient to an inappropriate unit or location, and care provision, such as incomplete or infrequent observation.

More than 90% of the organizations cited inadequate assessment as a root cause. More than 70% cited an unsafe environment of care. Approximately 65% cited insufficient staff orientation and training. More than 40% cited a communication failure, and approximately 30% cited the lack of vital information as root causes (see Figure 8-1, above). Nurses play a key role in the care of potentially suicidal individuals. A closer look at each root cause and prevention strategies nurses can use to reduce the likelihood of suicide follow.

Root Cause 1: Inadequate Assessment or Reassessment

Sentinel Event Example: Inadequate Assessment. *A man is admitted to the surgical unit of a hospital for evaluation and observation the night prior to his*

planned surgery to remove a cancerous lung tumor. He has had a biopsy and the diagnosis and plan are clear. Early that evening, the man kisses his wife "good night" and tells her he will see her in the morning. Later that evening, he gets himself ready for bed and turns off his light. At 10:30 PM, the nurse hears a very loud crash coming from the man's room. She hurries into the room, notes that the window has been shattered and that the man is no longer in the room. She runs to the window and sees the patient six stories below, lying face down. Security personnel, nurses arriving for the night shift, and visitors have responded and are summoning help. The man is transported to the emergency department where he is pronounced dead.

This example illustrates the danger of inadequate assessment. As mentioned earlier, inadequate assessment is the most frequently identified root cause of inpatient suicides. The purpose of *assessment* is to obtain appropriate and necessary information about each care recipient at times of entry into or transition within a health care setting or service. The information is used to match an individual's need with the appropriate setting, care level, and intervention. The purpose of *suicide assessment* is to identify individuals at increased risk for suicide, and to obtain clinical information relevant to their treatment planning. Periodic reassessment assures ongoing monitoring of suicide risk over time.

The Joint Commission requires organizations to have an assessment procedure for the early detection of problems that are life-threatening.

An initial screening, based on demographic characteristics of the individual and clinical and psychological indicators, provides the information necessary to determine whether suicide assessment is warranted. Although suicide risk is commonly not considered individuals who come into the acute care setting for medical or surgical reasons, the example above indicates that suicide risk must be considered with all care recipients.

Nursing assessments should consider the individual's perception of his or her disease and the plan of treatment. Cancer patients often are despondent. They may see their cancer diagnosis as a long slow death sentence that ultimately will sap their families' resources. Hence, the psychosocial portion of the assessment should be thoroughly completed. As surgical nurses would generally attest, physical assessment is well addressed in initial and ongoing assessment. The patient is physically prepared for the procedure, his or her vital signs are appropriate to allow the procedure, the necessary intravenous lines have been started, and the sites have been marked to assure surgery of the correct side, site, or limb. As a counterpart, the psychosocial assessment should address the individual's understanding of his or her disease and answer such questions as: Who does the individual live with? What are his or her expec-

tations of the planned surgery? What does he or she feel will be the impact on his or her life and that of the family?

Pastoral care is an integral part of the health care equation for many individuals. The nursing assessment includes specific queries about the care recipient's spirituality and the strengths that the person draws from religion and culture. Identification of the individual's cultural and spiritual needs is an important tool for the nurse in health care settings. These needs often provide insight into an individual's psychosocial status.

Nurses who perform a thorough and insightful assessment of the individual's psychological state prior to surgery may get a sense that the person is unhappy, nervous, and perhaps depressed. Referral of such a care recipient to a professional in psychology or psychiatry prior to surgery based on such an observation would at very least improve the individual's level of comfort and might avert a more serious outcome such as in the case of the man with lung cancer.

Clinicians must determine whether the individual presents low, moderate, or high suicide risk. Many organizations have compiled lists of common clues, danger signs, or risk factors that indicate a potentially suicidal individual and the need to seek professional help for suicide assessment and intervention. A list of commonly cited suicide risk factors appears in Sidebar 8-1, above.

SIDEBAR 8-2. SUICIDE SCREENING QUESTIONS FOR AN INITIAL ASSESSMENT

The following questions represent a sampling of possible suicide screening questions:

- Have you had thoughts of death or of killing yourself? What were they?
- What did you think about doing to yourself?
- Are you currently thinking about killing yourself?

- What are your thoughts on how, when and where you would do this?
- Have you attempted suicide in the past? What did you do?
- Has a close friend or anyone in the family committed suicide?
- Has anyone in the family ever been treated for depression or emotional illness?
- Have you tried to hurt yourself? If so, how?

Organizations must ensure that all care recipients are asked whether they have recently or in the past considered or attempted suicide. Thoughts of suicide (suicide ideation) as well as actual attempts are factors that significantly increase suicide risk and *must* be taken seriously.

Nurses need to be thorough in the assessment of the potential "lethality" of all individuals who are admitted to the health care organization, particularly the person with depression. It is not unusual for an individual to be admitted to a psychiatric unit in the middle of the night. In many hospitals, particularly small rural hospitals, a psychiatrist may not be available. Many individuals attempt suicide within the first few hours in the organization. Reliance on a pact with the individual that suicide will not be attempted is not adequate (see sentinel event example under Root Cause 2).

A true assessment of the lethality of the individual's suicidal ideation or potential must be conducted. This can be accomplished only with adequate historical information and is most productive if the organization has established clinical criteria to determine the degree to which intent in the individual's threats would lead to an attempt. Criteria will include the number of previous suicidal episodes, how they have been manifested, and what information can be obtained that would suggest that an individual might or might not attempt suicide. The influence of illicit substances is extremely important as well.

Proper assessment involves routinely asking individuals about their recent and past suicidal thoughts, feelings and plans. Asking the suicide ("S") question—"Have you ever had thoughts of killing yourself?"—is the direct way to ask the question to detect suicide risk. Yet, the question frequently is an uncomfortable one for staff members and may go unasked during initial and ongoing assessments. Compounding this, care recipients may be reluctant without a prompt to raise thoughts and feelings about suicide due to their own discomfort about the subject. Possible "S" questions to ask during an initial assessment appear in Sidebar 8-2, above.

Paul Quinnett, PhD, and his colleagues at Greentree Behavioral Health in Spokane, Washington, suggest asking the "S" question while obtaining background and family history for mental illness, substance abuse, and depression and mood disorders. In their suicide risk reduction program for hospitals,[10] they write, "The "S" question can be asked as follows, 'Has anyone in your family been depressed or seen a psychiatrist or counselor? Has anyone ever threatened, made an attempt or committed suicide?' This can then be followed by, 'Have you ever experienced thoughts of death or suicide or have you ever heard voices telling you to kill yourself?'" The only way *not* to ask the question, according to Quinnett, is phrasing it in a manner such as, "You're not thinking about suicide, are you?" This increases the individual's anxiety and sets up a negative response.

At the Warren Grant Magnuson Clinical Center of the National Institutes of Health in Bethesda, Maryland, each individual is assessed for self-harm and suicide potential within an hour of admission or risk identification in units or clinics. According to nursing department guidelines approved by Kathryn Lothschuetz Montgomery, RN, PhD, CNAA, associate director for nursing, nursing assessment includes thoughts of suicide (both active and passive), current suicidal intent, existence of a specific plan, availability of means to follow through with the plan, elopement potential, prior history of suicidal intent or previous suicide attempts, risk factors, and inadequate support system.[11]

"Organizations tend to make assessment errors at two points in the continuum of care: the first is soon after the individual is admitted and the second is when the person is starting to look and act better, showing sudden signs of improvement," says S. Virginia Knight, RN, PhD, a behavioral health care surveyor for the Joint Commission. "The new patient figures out how to commit suicide before the staff really gets a feel for him or her; the seemingly improved individual may be improved only because he or she has developed a suicide plan and medications have kicked in, providing the energy and focus to actually act on the plan," says Knight.

Jill Egger, RN, MSEd, Joint Commission sentinel event specialist, recommends that organizations treat sudden shifts of behavior as a red flag indicating the need for in-depth suicide assessment. These shifts are short-lasting and purposefully misleading clinical improvements. She suggests not leaving new patients alone, particularly those for whom little information is available on admissions. John Fishbeck, associate director of the Joint Commission's Department of Standards, recommends thorough assessment of the care recipient before any passes or outings are approved. "If the staff has any worries about the individual's safety, the person should not be allowed to leave the facility," says Fishbeck.

Prevention Strategies

Screen all admissions for suicide ideation. Nurses can be involved in developing and implementing an assessment tool that will effectively screen individuals for suicidal thoughts, gestures, and attempts. All individuals should be asked the "S" question. All staff, including nurses, should ask the individual about suicide as sensitively as possible, avoiding use of any words or statements that could seem judgmental. Research indicates that talking about suicidal thoughts provides relief for the care recipient.

Regularly review screening and assessment tools. The nursing staff should routinely review the effectiveness of assessment and screening tools. The initial assessment tool should serve as a screen, which, when tied into a scoring mechanism, triggers an in-depth behavioral assessment for individuals who receive an at-risk screening score. Staff may think that review and analysis of a tool used for the past three years are not necessary. However, this is not the case. Tools must be tested at regular intervals. Unfortunately, the tools used in many organizations have been designed only to meet regulatory requirements rather than to obtain data that will assist caregivers in providing appropriate care. Well-designed tools recognize that nurses need to apply critical thinking skills to the assessment rather than rote obedience.

When testing nursing assessment tools, nurses should ask, "What happens with the data that are collected during the assessment? If a care recipient indicates that he or she is 'sad' about his or her health status, or 'worried' and 'preoccupied' with the impact of the disease and the planned treatment on his or her family and on family resources, who receives such information and what do they do with it?" Some interventions that should be put in place based on specific assessment data are easy to recognize. For example, an overweight man weighing 283 pounds should be referred to a dietician for diet instruction. A woman with a new gait disturbance should be evaluated by a physical therapist. Psychological signs pointing to suicide risk are much more subtle but, when identified, could also trigger an applicable algorithm for intervention.

Should the individual who appears to have difficulty with his diagnosis and treatment plan be referred to the psychiatrist? Would the person

---

SIDEBAR 8-3. SITUATIONS REQUIRING SUICIDE RISK ASSESSMENT AND DOCUMENTATION

- On admission
- When the individual exhibits suicidal behavior or expresses suicidal thoughts
- When a clinical or behavioral change occurs

- Prior to granting increased privileges or a pass
- When the individual returns from a pass
- Prior to discharge

---

benefit from a visit by a member of the pastoral care staff? Finally, is there reason to believe that the individual may take drastic action related to his or her feelings that would have devastating consequences? Nurses conducting a comprehensive initial assessment that includes physical and psychological indicators can address these questions. Using appropriate tools, nurses can identify subtle nuances in the individual's psyche during times of understandably great stress.

Be a good listener and ensure that you obtain complete information. Active listening is critical during the assessment process as are complete answers. If necessary, the nurse assessing the care recipient should ask him or her to provide more information and give the person time to respond. Individuals who are experiencing psychological stress about treatment may need more prompting for complete answers and time to respond.

Reassess during high-risk times of transition. Because change is stressful for many care recipient, times of transition are high-risk periods for suicide in a 24-hour care setting. Hence, leaders must ensure that staff reassess care recipients at these times. As mentioned earlier, the period occurring shortly after an individual is admitted is a high-risk time. The individual may still have a viable suicide plan and the intent to implement it. In addition, suicide risk is especially high at the time of discharge. The transition from inpatient to outpatient care often is problematic because, for example, the individual may be anxious about returning to an unsheltered and non-supportive environment.

Thorough reassessment prior to granting an individual a pass or increased privileges is criti-

cal due to the high frequency of suicide while individuals are out on passes or authorized visits. Nurses and other staff should assess what support systems are available to the individual on a pass. If support from family or friends is not available, if family will increase the individual's stress, anger, or other adverse emotions, or if the nurse has any worries about the individual's safety, the person should not be allowed to leave the facility.

In addition, the care recipient should be reassessed on return from passes or other special privileges. The stress of visiting an unchanged home environment that may have precipitated the crisis or negative interactions with others during the pass can rekindle suicidal ideation. Also, passes may permit depressed individuals access to the means of completing suicide that are not available in health care settings. Passes also could permit access to illegal substances that could affect the individual's mood and hence, suicidal intent. See Sidebar 8-3, above, for a summary of situations requiring suicide risk assessment and documentation.

Advocate for a uniform approach to both assessment and documentation of suicidality. A uniform, standardized approach to suicide assessment and documentation increases the likelihood that the right clinical questions will be asked and relevant information obtained.[12] "If an inpatient service uses a standardized assessment form, however, there should be a clear understanding that the form does not substitute for clinical judgment, and whatever uniform approach is used, adequate opportunity should be left for the clinician to make additional comments or observations," notes Gary Jacobson.[12]

Root Cause 2: Unsafe Environment of Care

Sentinel Event Example: Unsafe Environmental Factors. *The police bring a 50-year-old man to a small, rural community hospital at 12:30 AM. The man had been in the town "lock-up" since 7:00 PM following an altercation with his girlfriend. While in police custody, the man had become progressively more despondent and had made gestures suggesting that he wanted to commit suicide.*

Following evaluation in the emergency department, the man is admitted to the 15-bed acute psychiatric unit. The nurse on duty assesses the man and conducts an interview. The nurse asks him if he currently has or has had suicidal thoughts. Appearing remorseful, the man indicates that he had thoughts of suicide earlier that evening and that he had made threats in the police department so that he could get out of jail. He tells the nurse that he is no longer contemplating suicide and that he does not have a suicide plan. The man signs an agreement that he will not hurt himself. The nurse is very much relieved and shows the man to his room, placing him on a 20-minute observation schedule and informing him that he would be visited by the unit's psychiatrist in the morning.

A mental health worker, who is the only other employee on this unit, makes rounds about 25 minutes later. The worker finds the man sitting on the toilet, slumped forward, hanging from the water supply pipe of the toilet. The man had torn his T-shirt into strips of sufficient length to tie around his neck and the flush mechanism on the toilet water supply pipe. The worker calls a code but resuscitative efforts are unsuccessful.

Environmental factors contributed to this man's suicide completion. A pipe was available for his use in hanging himself. Multiple environmental opportunities, beyond the obvious, present themselves to the individual inclined to carry out suicide. The organization in the example above might already have replaced shower curtain rods with breakaway rods, and shower heads with beveled or breakaway shower heads, as recommended by experts. However, staff failed to identify other environmental hazards, such as the toilet's water supply pipe. Many toilets do not have fill tanks, but have high pressure flush hardware from which an individual can hang him or herself. Some organizations

have recognized this problem and have recessed the plumbing into the wall behind the toilet with only a push button exposed. Disability grab bars present another hazard because individuals can wrap string, a belt, or an article of clothing around them to commit a suicide.

Prevention Strategies

Be knowledgeable about environmental hazards and advocate for their removal. Nurses need to be aware of areas and elements of the environment that represent an opportunity for individuals intent on committing suicide. The removal of environmental hazards is particularly important for the individual who has clear signs of suicidality with significant lethality. Under such circumstances, frequent evaluation or even one-on-one observation will be implemented. Nevertheless, a general awareness of how individuals could carry out suicide is important knowledge for nurses and particularly psychiatric nurses to possess.

Since hanging is the most common method of inpatient suicide, a popular myth about hanging should be addressed. David M. Sine, consultant to the National Association of Psychiatric Health Systems, mentions that a widely pervasive misconception of what it takes to hang yourself still exists in modern society. "Someone intent on suicide doesn't need to figure out a way to suspend his or her whole body weight. All they have to do is wrap something around their neck, attach it to something solid, and lean forward, even from a kneeling position. It takes much less weight than many think," explains Sine.[13]

Door hinges, door knobs, non-breakaway bathroom fixtures, exposed lighting fixtures, closet poles, metal hangers, and other potential environmental hazards should be removed, whenever possible. Sidebar 8-4, page 98, presents other recommendations regarding the environment of care. Understanding the threats in the environment and completing a thorough assessment of the individual's intent to commit suicide provides a critical opportunity for caregivers in psychiatric units and facilities to implement appropriate observation and control

SIDEBAR 8-4. ENVIRONMENT OF CARE RECOMMENDATIONS

Although most experts agree that it is not possible to "suicide-proof" any space, the following recommendations can remove the most obvious environmental hazards.

- Identify and remove or replace non-breakaway hardware in bathing facilities.
- Assure that existing breakaway hardware has been appropriately weight tested.
- Redesign, retrofit or introduce security measures (for example, locking mechanisms, patient monitors, and alarms).

- Keep the care recipient's personal laundry facilities closed and locked and implement systems to monitor individuals who need to do their laundry.
- Remove plastic liners from trash cans to prevent asphyxiation by packing the oropharynx or placing bags over the head.
- Shorten the nurse call pull cords in bathrooms so they cannot be used for strangulation.

measures. Individuals who are at risk should be moved to areas where continuous observation can occur until lethality of suicidality has abated. Staffing should be adjusted to consider environmental hazards that cannot immediately be addressed. When substantive changes to the environment are not possible, close observation of the care recipient is the best nursing strategy.

Assess individual's environment of care and make appropriate adjustments. While experts emphasize that high quality care is the most effective means to reduce the risk of suicide, organization leaders should examine the care environments to ensure that they are as safe and secure as possible. Leaders are required to ensure the design of a safe, accessible, effective, and efficient environment of care that meets the needs of individuals served. The potentially suicidal individual presents significant challenges in this regard. Management plans must address safety and security and such plans must be implemented. Organizations must meet the challenge of providing a safe environment of care while maintaining individual rights, such as the right to privacy, dignity, and a therapeutic environment.

Nurses do not always have control over needed changes to the existing care environment. However, they can assess an individual's needs and, if possible, adjust where the individual is cared for in the existing environment. For example, geriatric patients in psychiatric units

of community hospitals often need grab bars in bathrooms and showers to hold onto while toileting and attending to personal hygiene. However, younger individuals without a physical disability who are deemed suicidal might use the same devices to attempt suicide by hanging. Therefore, it is critical for nurses to assess the environment to which the individual is assigned and adjust the person's location or the level of observation accordingly.

Root Cause 3: Insufficient Staff Orientation, Training, and Competence Assessment and Inadequate Staffing

Sentinel Event Example: Inadequate Staffing Level.
A 28-year-old man is combative on a psychiatric unit and requires restraint. After becoming more subdued, the man is placed into seclusion because there is insufficient staff to continuously monitor his behavior. In seclusion, he is alone for long enough to remove the draw string from his gym shorts, tie a slip noose around his neck, and strangle himself.

Sentinel Event Example: Insufficient Training.
An 80-year-old man in a long term care facility appears to be complying with his medication therapy. Two times each day, a nurse delivers his medication dose to his room. However, he fakes swallowing them and moves them with his tongue into the space between the cheek and lower or upper gums (the "buccal gutter"). Once the nurse leaves his room, he removes the medications from his mouth and stores the

pills in a hiding place in his clothes drawer. Eight days later, he takes all of the medications at once, causing a fatal arrhythmia and death by overdose.

Staffing levels and the orientation and training of staff play a major role in an organization's effort to reduce suicide risk. In both of these examples, staffing, training, and appropriate observation of the care recipient are issues. An individual known to be suicidal should not be left alone in seclusion. In seclusion without proper observation by a staff member, this person is more likely to become disconnected and to realize that he or she has an opportunity to carry out suicide. In addition, staff in the first example were not aware of the fact that the man's shorts contained a drawstring that could be used for self harm. Clearly this staff needed education about suicide risk and how to advocate for adequate staff to care for individuals who are depressed and combative.

Some organizations may need to update their staffing models to ensure appropriate staff level and mix to meet care needs. Level and mix of staff caring for potentially suicidal individuals should be based on the acuity of the population. Experts differ regarding the staffing required for implementation of effective suicide precautions. Some now believe that the only truly effective precaution for high-risk individuals is one-on-one observation at no more than an arm's length distance. Organization leaders need to consider how to provide adequate staffing given the degree of risk with specific individuals. Additional mental health technicians or other staff members may be needed to observe care recipients on a busy psychiatric unit. Unfortunately, when a crisis presents itself in the middle of a shift, many departments respond by assigning a staff member from the unit to sit with the individual one-on-one. The staff person is not replaced and the unit continues to function with a staff shortage, which places other care recipients at risk.

Staff orientation and training are key to the proper assessment of suicidal risk and the prevention of suicide. At the completion of orientation, all staff members must demonstrate knowledge, skills, and competence sufficient to assume assigned responsibilities. Organization leaders must ensure that all nursing staff and all other staff with direct contact with care recipients receive education about the prevalence of suicide in health care settings. Too often, suicide "pacts" between care recipients and nurses are taken as gospel that the individual will not attempt to harm him or herself. Yet, all along, the individual is continuing to prepare for suicide in subtle ways that may not be recognized by a caregiver whose training or observation skills are inadequate. Nurses need to be aware of the practice of placing medications into the space between the teeth and the cheek, sometimes called "cheeking." Oral examination after a care recipient swallows medications may be a requisite for those who have been known to hide medications.

Nurses should receive education about the setting in which individuals will receive care. Individuals considered at risk for suicide will often be placed on a unit where movement or activity is restricted. These units will often have a higher patient-to-caregiver ratio. It is critical that nurses continue to receive education related to assessing care recipient needs so that nurses can advocate for the appropriate placement of the individual in the correct setting.

Orientation of new staff is crucial. No staff members should be allowed to work in care areas until they demonstrate a thorough understanding of all of the aspects of assessment and care of this patient population. Following orientation, the competence of the nurse in managing potentially suicidal individuals in crisis includes

- excellence in assessment skills to determine from the individual's level of agitation, despondency, and behavior that this is an individual in crisis. Sometimes a very calm and composed person has resolved to carry out a suicide.

- an understanding of the environment of care. If not all of the rooms have been made as free of hazards as possible, where should the individual be placed in the unit?

- an understanding of the individual's medication needs and when the individual should be medicated.

Competence must be assessed on a regular basis.

Prevention Strategies

Know suicide risk factors and categories of individuals at risk for suicide. Nurses must be knowledgeable about suicide risk factors and about at-risk individuals in their care. Nurses and caregivers in all health settings should be well trained in suicide risk and suicide prevention strategies. This is particularly important in behavioral settings. The mental health technician, psychiatric aide, social worker, counselor, psychologist, and nurse are all part of the team that will have constant or daily contact with the care recipient. Physicians also need to be continuously re-sensitized to evaluate suicidality in their interventional therapies. All staff should be aware that suicidal individuals do not always look and act the way staff expect suicidal individuals to act and look. For example, a suicidal individual may not be agitated and pacing the room or despondent and sitting motionless in a chair. A person having command hallucinations to kill him or herself may "look normal" and "act normally."

Nurses not comfortable with their level of skill and knowledge should request additional training. All nurses should be aware that psychological data obtained in the initial assessment might point toward suicidal ideation and should be followed up.

Ensure personal comfort level in caring for the suicidal individual. As a part of initial and ongoing training, nursing leaders should provide nursing staff with an opportunity to explore their feelings about caring for the suicidal individual. Many people are fearful of suicide and considerable training is necessary to increase comfort levels in talking about it. Nurses and other staff members may be afraid that if they mention suicide to a person, he or she will get the idea to kill him or herself. Education corrects this assumption. All nurses caring for the potentially suicidal individual should be trained in the philosophy of suicide prevention, the organization's approach to suicide risk reduction, the recognition of suicidal warning signs, and referral or communication procedures. Some training programs include structured role-playing in which nurses and other clinicians must elicit "hidden" risk factors during practice interviews.[10] Many organizations integrate role

playing of crisis situations in their crisis training modules. Crisis intervention training is expected for all nurses in care settings where care recipients may be combative and need restraint or seclusion.

Be familiar with and weigh issues related to care recipient's rights, age, and disability-specific needs for safety. There is a fine line between patient self-determination/patient rights and restriction of activity and freedom for safety reasons. Nursing staff should be well trained about appropriate interaction with the psychiatric patient. This education needs to be age specific and also address components of care recipient functionality. Addressing the suicidality of individuals who are mentally ill or developmentally disabled will present new and varied challenges. Care recipient rights during contraband searches need to be ensured. Nurses should assess possessions for their potential use in self injury. Sequestering belongings may be important. The care recipient may need hair dryers, cigarettes, cigarette lighters or matches, hair brushes, shampoo, and so forth only for short periods of time while in use.

Be knowledgeable about how to detect and remove contraband. Removal of items that might be dangerous to a suicidal individual is one of the most obvious yet key strategies in reducing suicide risk. Nurses must be well trained in implementing the organization's policies and procedures for the detection and removal of contraband. On admission to a behavioral health unit, individuals should be searched for dangerous items including belts, shoelaces, matches, lighters, sharp items, drugs, and weapons. Whenever the individual leaves the unit with a pass, he or she should be searched on return to the unit. Items from home that may seem innocent enough, such as a pair of walking shoes or sneakers, may have shoelaces that could be used for self injury. Individuals intent on self harm sometimes accumulate articles for a long time with the intent of using them for self-destructive purposes at some point. Nurses have to be aware of the items care recipients are receiving, storing, and sending.

Inform supervisor of unsafe staffing situations. Leaders must ensure that nurse supervisors are able to make and implement appropriate decisions about necessary staffing, including one-on-one staffing, if necessary. All nurses should report unsafe staffing situations through the channels established by organization policies and procedures.

Root Cause 4: Incomplete Caregiver Communication or Lack of Critical Information

Sentinel Event Example: Incomplete Communication Among Staff. *A 32-year-old man with a history of depression and suicidal ideation is admitted to the psychiatric unit of a community hospital. According to organization protocols, which apply to all care recipients independent of the severity of the individuals' illness, he is placed on intermittent observation and checked at 15-minute intervals. A mental health worker performs the checks, documenting his observations by placing a check mark by each care recipient's name on an observation checklist. The worker performs this function quickly every 15 to 25 minutes since there are other duties to perform. He is not aware of the man's at-risk-for-suicide status because staff performing the admissions assessment had not communicated this information.*

The worker's quick glance at the individuals in the common room verifies that all but one care recipient are present. The mental health worker places a check mark next to all but one of the names and asks the nursing staff where the missing man is. A nurse tells the worker that the man went back to his room to use the bathroom. Assuming that he had accounted for the missing man, the worker places a check mark next to the man's name. About 15 minutes later, the worker repeats the process. This time, the man still is not back in the common room. The mental health worker interrupts the activities session and asks one of the other care recipients to check on the missing patient. The other care recipient does so, and states "He is still in the bathroom." The worker places a check next to the man's name.

A nurse going by the man's room sees light coming from the bottom of the bathroom door and remembers that the patient in that room is at risk for suicide. She knocks on the bathroom door. Receiving no response, she goes to the common room to see if the man is involved in the activities session. She asks about the man's whereabouts. The mental health worker and

other patients chime in, "He is in the bathroom. He wasn't feeling well." The nurse runs back to the room, opens the bathroom door, and finds the man unresponsive on the floor. A code is called, but the man cannot be resuscitated.

Incomplete caregiver communication, inadequate information related to the care recipient, and inadequate observation are the issues in this example. The mental health worker was not aware of the man's at-risk status, and hence did not conduct appropriate checks. Some patients are on 15-minute checks for confusion and might be found wandering aimlessly up and down the corridor. Other patients might be on 15-minute checks because they are at risk for elopement. Still others, such as was the case with the man in this example, are checked at regular intervals because they are at risk for suicide. Incomplete communication among caregivers or the lack of vital information when needed can increase the risk of suicide. Inadequate observation, to be addressed in the next section, can do likewise.

The purpose of an interdisciplinary treatment planning process in all care settings is to assure that all caregivers are aware of each care recipient's needs so that care interventions can be collaboratively implemented by caregivers from a variety of disciplines. Communication provides the foundation for this process. If some caregivers are not adequately informed of an individual's needs, sentinel events can ensue. Transmission of data and information must be timely, accurate, and complete. The care recipient's clinical record must contain sufficient information to support clinical decisions. Past suicide attempts, triggers that may influence behaviors, and any recent changes that have occurred in the person's life must be identified. The review of data related to admission to other organizations may play a key role in identifying the care recipient at risk for suicide.

The accurate and timely sharing of this information among caregivers is crucial to providing the best care in the safest possible environment. Caregiver communication and information transfer were severely lacking in the previous example. As key caregivers, nurses can implement proactive strategies to enhance communication and information transfer, and thereby reduce suicide risk.

Prevention Strategies

Help ensure complete information transfer on admission. An organization's admission policies and procedures should minimize the occurrence of admission of individuals for whom medical and psychiatric histories are unavailable. When information on admission is insufficient, nursing and other staff can not ensure the individual's safety. Nurses can follow up to obtain missing information.

Document and communicate key assessment findings. Once the initial admission assessment has occurred, findings need to be thoroughly documented and properly communicated by the nursing and other clinical staff to appropriate colleagues. On occasion, staff may complete the assessment within the required time frame, but then forget to include the material in the clinical record or communicate significant findings to appropriate colleagues. Nurses can help ensure that documentation happens within the required time frame and that the documents are signed and validated by the physician. The information cannot be waiting on a transcription line somewhere: it has to be available to caregivers to aide decision making. For example, if assessment findings indicate that an individual is at high risk for suicide, staff must be informed immediately in order to implement line-of-sight or even arm's length, one-on-one, observation procedures.

Help ensure complete information transfer during provision of care. Thorough communication among the nurses and other staff members involved in the care of a potentially suicidal individual is a critical factor in reducing the risk of suicide. Information about changes in an individual's behavior, however small, may signal a trend and must be communicated to caregivers on the current and next shift. For example, if a person's behavior improves dramatically and he or she starts cleaning his or her room, participating in groups sessions, and so forth, staff should document and communicate these behaviors from one shift to another. Behavior such as slowly giving away possessions to other patients or having

family members take articles home can be signs of renewed suicidal ideation. Documentation via written notes in the chart or verbal reports should prompt a reassessment of the individual for the availability of a suicide plan. All high-risk thoughts, feelings, and behaviors exhibited or expressed by an individual must be clearly communicated to other caregivers.

Thorough information transfer must occur during all phases of care. Communication at time of shift change is particularly important. The oncoming shift needs to be aware of issues related to specific aspects of each individual's care. For example, on a behavioral health care unit, nursing staff should report to oncoming staff any change in an individual's behavior that warrants watching during the next shift. Communication of changes to physicians who may not be on the unit at all times is also important. Through initial and revised orders, physicians specify the interventions required to care for each individual. Lack of communication regarding care recipient changes to all members of the team can be devastating.

Help ensure complete information transfer prior to discharge. Because discharge represents a transition for the individual—a high-risk time for suicide—the thorough transfer of information at this point and thorough communication are particularly critical. Nurses often play a critical role at this point. The individual and family or significant others should be informed about what might increase the risk of the return of suicidality, such as discontinuation of medications and noncompliance with the treatment plan. They also should be informed about ongoing treatment needs, community resources, and how to access emergency services after discharge.

Root Cause 5: Inadequate Care Planning or Care Provision

Following initial assessment of the potentially suicidal individual, organization staff develop a care plan tailored to meet the individual's needs. As the individual receives care, he or she is reassessed for suicide risk and the care plan is revised as appropriate to treatment goals and results. Leaders must ensure that the care plan fully reflects the individual's assessment and

SIDEBAR 8-5. SUICIDE RISK LEVELS

- *Lowest risk:* Individual expresses no thoughts of death.
- *Low risk:* Individual expresses thoughts of death, but not by suicide.
- *Moderate risk:* Individual expresses suicidal thoughts without having considered the specific method.
- *High risk:* Individual expresses suicidal thoughts and has determined a specific plan.

reassessment findings and the care plans vary by risk levels. Sidebar 8-5, above, describes risk categories used by many organizations. These risk levels then tie to specific treatment protocols. For example, a high risk individual, like the man described in the example under Root Cause 4 (pages 88–89), would be placed on continuous observation. Level or risk categories, determined during an assessment, should correlate with level of care decisions, determined during the care planning process. In turn, level of care decisions should identify the specific suicide precaution level appropriate to each individual. Leaders must establish clear policies on monitoring levels and ensure that these are reflected in policies and procedure manuals and are effectively communicated to the staff.

The care plan must be developed and implemented by all members of the care team. The plan must address the care recipient's specific needs and the multidisciplinary interventions to meet such needs. If the care plan calls for observation, for example, the observation level must be delineated clearly so that none of the caregivers have questions about what such observation entails.

Nurses play a key role in the care planning and care provision processes. As the professionals most often providing round-the-clock care, nurses often coordinate the planning process and implementation of care interventions, whether on a one-time or ongoing basis. Too often, care planning is conducted in a perfunctory manner, solely to meet regulatory or accreditation requirements. In all care settings, a well developed plan is one that becomes the guideline for the individual's care. Nurses collect data related to the individual's response to treatment and interventions outlined in the plan and report these back to the team so that appropriate changes to the plan can be made, as necessary.

The treatment plan must address as a primary function the individual's safety. The plan provides the basis for appropriate observation of the individual in the care setting and for participation in therapeutic activities. Revision of the plan may be required when changes are noted in the individual's condition or behavior. Nurses help to ensure that all caregivers receive appropriate information regarding plan revisions.

Care planning problems have been identified as one of the root causes of many of the suicides reviewed by the Joint Commission. Such problems include assignment of the individual to an inappropriate unit or location, or placement of the suicidal individual in seclusion with restraints as standard operating procedure.

Prevention Strategies

Help ensure completion of all assessments prior to initiation of care planning. To ensure appropriate care, all disciplines' assessments must be up to date and completed prior to the initiation of effective care planning. Nurses can help to identify whether any assessments are missing. Individuals may provide different responses to queries related to their potential suicidality. A nurse may be able to obtain a piece of information that a psychologist or social worker could not, or vice versa.

Actively participate in the care planning process and communicate care plan details to involved caregivers. Nurses should actively participate in care planning and help to ensure adequate documentation of the interdisciplinary care plan and its dissemination to all disciplines and caregivers involved. This involves communicating about the tasks expected of assistive caregivers, such as mental health workers, nursing assistants, psychiatric technicians, recreation therapists, and others. Nurses may need to communicate directly with the mental health technician at the beginning of each shift, for example, to reiterate the need for close observation depending on the behavior the individual displays. Nurses also communicate the tenets of the care plan to the care recipient. A care recipient needs to buy into his or her plan of care if results are to be achieved.

Help to ensure implementation of the appropriate observation level. Nurses can ensure implementation of the suicide precautions written by a physician or other clinician specifying a level of surveillance of the individual by the nursing or assistive staff. Precautions involve constant or intermittent observation or some gradation thereof.

Communicate the need to change an individual's observation level. Just as choosing the initial observation level requires considerable thought, so does increasing or decreasing the monitoring level. In some organizations, nurses, social workers, or others are allowed to implement a stricter, more protective monitoring level, while orders from a licensed independent practitioner are required for a decreased monitoring level. Evaluation and feedback from the nurse observer team are critical to changing monitoring levels.

Help to ensure thorough implementation of observation policies and procedures. Leaders must ensure thorough implementation of observation procedures and monitor staff performance of such procedures. The mental health worker described in the example under Root Cause 4 (pages 88–89) did not complete observation procedures as per organization policy. Nurses can help identify the occurrence of incomplete observations and take necessary steps to address the situation.

Ensure proper supervision during high-risk activities. Leaders must ensure that supervision is ade-

quate during high-risk activities. Nurses should be aware that what often appear to be low-risk activities, such as the individual taking a shower or using the toilet, are in fact high-risk times for suicide. As mentioned previously, a large proportion of suicides take place in the bathroom. While nurses and other staff observing a high-risk individual on a one-on-one basis may wish to give him or her privacy in the bathroom, doing so does not provide adequate observation to ensure safety. If an individual expresses suicidal thoughts, nurses should be alert to use of tools during activities (especially occupational therapy), objects that might be picked up when escorting the individual outside, and signs that the individual is storing up medication.[14]

Concluding Comment

Suicides by care recipients in 24-hour care facilities represent a tragic sentinel event. Nurses can proactively prevent such occurrences by working with other health care team members to ensure adequate care recipient assessment and reassessment, a safe environment of care, proper orientation, training and competence assessment, sufficient staffing, complete communication, accurate and timely information transfer, thorough care planning, and high quality care provision.

References

1. AAS: *1998 National Suicide Statistics and Facts.* American Association of Suicidology, June 1999. (Available on the Web at *www.suicidology.org.*)

2. Busch KA, et al: Clinical features of inpatient suicide. *Psych Annals* 23(5):256–262, 1993.

3. Farberow NL: Guidelines to suicide prevention in the hospital. In Shneidman ES, Farberow NL, Litman RL (eds): *The Psychology of Suicide: A Clinician's Guide to Evaluation and Treatment.* Northvale, NJ: J. Aronson, 1994.

4. Blumenthal SJ: Suicide: A guide to risk factors, assessment, and treatment of suicidal patients. *Med Clin North Am* 72(4):937–971, 1988.

5. Jacobson G: The inpatient management of suicidality. In Jacobs DG (ed): *The Harvard Medical School Guide to Suicide Assessment and Intervention.* San Francisco: Jossey-Bass, 1999, p 383.

6. Litman RE: Suicide prevention in a treatment setting. *Suicide Life Threat Behav* 25(1):134–142, 1995.

7. Busch KA, Clark DC, Kravitz HM: Clinical features of inpatient suicide. *Psychiatr Annals* 23(5):256–262, 1993.

8. Cardell R, Horton-Deutsch SL: A model for assessment of inpatient suicide potential. *Arch Psychiatr Nurs* 8(6):366–372, 1994.

9. Joint Commission: Inpatient suicides: Recommendations for prevention. *Sentinel Event Alert* issue 7, Nov 6, 1998.

10. Cardell R, Quinnett P, Bratcher K: *QPRT-H Suicide Risk Management Inventory-Hospital Version.* Spokane, WA: Cardell, Quinnett, and Bratcher, 1999.

11. Joint Commission: Asking the "suicide question": Assess thoroughly and often to reduce risk. *Joint Commission Benchmark* 1(6):1–3, Aug 1999.

12. Jacobson G: The inpatient management of suicidality. In Jacobs DG (ed): *The Harvard Medical School Guide to Suicide Assessment and Intervention.* San Francisco: Jossey-Bass, 1999, p 386.

13. Personal communication with David Sine, Jun 1999.

14. Reynolds DK, Farberow NL: *Suicide: Inside and Out.* Berkeley, CA: University of California Press, 1976, pp 191–193.

Chapter 9:

Preventing Treatment Delays

Organizationwide performance of tests, procedures, treatment, or service must be effective, continuous with other care and care providers, safe, efficient, respectful of the care recipient, and rendered in a timely manner. *Treatment delay* occurs when any factor is not provided to the care recipient in a time frame required to meet his or her care needs. In the best case, such delay may result in inconveniencing the individual and his or her family. In the worst case, the delay may result in death or serious physical or psychological injury.

The systems established by health care organizations for providing care and services and the ability of staff within the organization to move care recipients through the health care process are foremost in maintaining timely care. Organization leaders, including nurse leaders, must identify the needs of the populations served and establish the spectrum of care services that will meet those needs in a timely manner that is consistent with the organization's mission. The system of care for individuals served by the organization includes the following phases:

- Access to the care system;
- Admission to the care system;
- Care within the system; and
- Discharge from the care system.

Many factors associated with each of these phases can impede the timely completion of care. Nurses are integrally involved in each of the phases.

Cause for Concern

Data from the Joint Commission's Sentinel Event database, including nearly 1,100 sentinel events

reviewed by the organization from January 1995 through June 2001, indicate that delay in treatment accounted for 5.4% of sentinel events, representing the fifth most common type of sentinel event reviewed by the organization. Root causes of treatment delay include

- inadequate communication among caregivers;
- insufficient staff orientation and training or insufficient staffing;
- inadequate care recipient assessment;
- inadequate information management; and
- faulty equipment or environment of care problems.

A closer look at each root cause will help to identify strategies nurses can use to reduce the likelihood of treatment delay-related deaths and injuries.

Root Cause 1: Inadequate Communication Among Caregivers

Sentinel Event Example: Communication Problems. *A frail, elderly woman with a fast and thready pulse is admitted to the hospital from a long term care facility. The admitting physician is worried that the woman's dosage of digoxin, one of several cardiac medications the woman is receiving, may not have been sufficient to strengthen her heartbeat and prevent pulmonary edema. The physician orders a digoxin level to be drawn with the afternoon laboratory values. The nurse misses the order on the admission order form and does not include an order for a digoxin level on the slip provided to the laboratory phlebotomist drawing the woman's blood.*

The physician visits the woman during rounds that night. She notes rales during ascultation of the woman's breath sounds and that the woman appears to be more congested. The physician makes a mental note to check the digoxin level since the woman's pulse is weak and fast. When reviewing the woman's clinical record, the physician does not see the results of the ordered digoxin level and assumes that it was an oversight on his part. She orders another digoxin level to be drawn in the morning and also orders 40 mg of Lasix. The physician did not order digoxin to be given when the woman arrived earlier in the day and she did not order digoxin to be administered when she saw her later that night.

The nurse caring for the woman on the evening shift removes the orders for the blood draw in the morning and does not review the record for outstanding orders for previous blood specimens. The nurse on the day shift when the woman was admitted also did not review the pending laboratory tests, which would have indicated the fact that the digoxin level was not drawn. The patient receives 40mg of Lasix and appears to be breathing a little more easily. The report to the night shift nurse states that the woman appeared to have some labored respiration which resolved with Lasix.

At about 2:00 AM in the morning, the woman becomes very short of breath and is clearly in pulmonary edema. The nurse on the night shift telephones the resident on call to come visit the woman. The resident evaluates the woman and reviews the record, noting that a digoxin level was ordered when the woman was admitted and that the results were not in the record. She asks the nurse why the results were not obtained. The night nurse calls the laboratory. Laboratory staff acknowledge that they did not receive a slip for the earlier draw but that the woman is on the morning roster for digoxin levels. They suggest that if the physician is concerned, the physician ask for the results "Stat." They indicate that digoxin levels cannot be run on the off-shift hours.

The resident appears satisfied with that explanation and orders more Lasix, reduces the IV fluid volume rate, and leaves the unit. The woman diureses, improves slightly, and breathes through the night. The levels are drawn the next morning, but the results are not requested "Stat." The day shift nurse does not follow up on the status of the results, which indicate insufficient digoxin levels. The results are filed in the woman's record without action.

At about noon, the woman experiences cardiac arrest and cannot be resuscitated. The attending physician is informed that the woman has expired. He comes to the nurses station to fill out the death certificate. Reviewing the woman's record, he realizes that the first digoxin level was not drawn. The value from the morning draw indicates that the cause of death is directly related to the lack of digoxin. The physician calls the hospital's risk manager to express concern about treatment delays.

Adequate and effective communication among caregivers is key to the provision of high quality care and the prevention of sentinel events related to treatment delays. In this example, communication was inadequate on a number of fronts. The physician should have ordered a hold on the Digoxin dose for that morning until the levels were received and then suggested a call for advice on appropriate dosing. The physician might have left dosing parameters for the nurse to follow dependent on the levels of Digoxin in the woman's blood. In this case, the nurse would have been able to make an appropriate determination of the dose or if the dose needed to be withheld and the level reevaluated. The night nurse had a responsibility to communicate the pending laboratory results that would impact the woman's medication. The day nurse had a responsibility to review the pending laboratory results and to adjust the woman's medication schedule. The day nurse could have held the Digoxin until the lab values were received and then called the physician for a dose adjustment. Laboratories must flag unusual or significant test results in a manner that will draw attention to the findings.

Too often, staff will seek out over-simplistic solutions to such communication failures, for example, by having all individuals receive Digoxin in the afternoon when lab test results generally are available. If the nursing staff does not understand the rationale of this practice, errors may occur. Leaders need to involve nursing staff in devising systems that enhance effective communication about care recipients.

Prevention Strategies

Ensure effective communication of information related to care recipient needs from one shift to the next. Nurses need to establish and implement workable communication systems to transmit information from one caregiver to the next. In-person shift reports and written documentation are most effective. Tape-recorded reports, although commonly used as a back-up mechanism, do not provide the opportunity for the oncoming shift to ask questions of the previous shift. It is imperative that the nurse beginning to care for an individual receives *all* of the required information at the beginning of the shift. Nurses can document critical elements on forms developed to capture key information that must be communicated to the next shift. Such forms help to ensure that the nurse remembers to communicate necessary information during the verbal report.

Respond promptly and appropriately to critical information received from other disciplines. Nursing staff must know how to appropriately "process" information critical to care recipient safety and other outcomes. For example, in the scenario provided above, the nurse should know to call the woman's physician with the test results. This assumes the nurse's competence in understanding the appropriate levels of Digoxin in the blood. Nurses can help to ensure that information received from laboratories effectively uses a system to flag abnormal results. A system of "panic-value" reporting must be implemented.

Root Cause 2: Insufficient Staff Orientation and Training or Insufficient Staffing

Sentinel Event Example: Insufficient Orientation. *A 60-year-old woman goes to an ambulatory care clinic to receive her annual physical from her long-time physician. The physician gives the woman a prescription for an annual mammogram, which she schedules for two weeks later. Following the mammogram, the woman is informed that there are "problems" with the test and that she will hear from her physician's office. A week later, a nurse in the physician's office calls the woman and informs her that additional mammogram views are required. The nurse does not express the physician's wish that the tests be done immediately nor that there is a potential health problem. Required to perform extra duties because of short staffing, the nurse files the X-ray reports in the woman's medical record rather than in the proper file for tests requiring follow up.*

The woman does not forget the need for a follow-up mammogram and calls the physician's office to ascertain whether a repeat mammogram has been ordered. Another office employee assumes that if the woman did not get a call from the physician directly, the woman has nothing to worry about and should relax. Lacking assertiveness, the woman does not question the employee's answer, nor tell her about the nurse's call, and attempts to think no more about it.

Several weeks later, the woman calls the physician's office again, noting that she can feel a hard lump in her breast and mentioning that it hurts. The physician tells her to come into the office right away. Upon review of her record, the physician finds the results and orders another mammogram with needle localization "Stat." The woman has the test, which identifies a change in the size of a nodule from a previous mammogram. This requires an immediate biopsy which is positive. Subsequent surgery reveals that the cancer has metastasized.

This example illustrates the critical link between staff training, staffing levels, and the provision of timely treatment. All types of health care organizations frequently struggle with the challenge of maintaining adequate staffing in times of increasing care loads. Staff positions may be reevaluated and staff members cross-trained to work in multiple areas. The nurse in the example above had been trained in another physician's office to file all results, abnormal as well as normal, in the clinical record.

All practitioners have preferences for the particular way that data, including test results, are processed. In the woman's case, the newly cross-trained nurse did not process the report following the practitioner's procedure. Cross-trained staff must be thoroughly trained in procedures and protocols and ask questions about procedures to use when there is an unusual situation like abnormal test findings. Organizations should also consider standardizing the procedure used to process data, including test results, so that all practitioners follow the same procedure. This would free nurses from having to recall the different preferences of each practitioner.

Insufficient staffing levels also could have contributed to the delay in the woman's treatment. Care areas must be adequately staffed to assess and care for individuals. Staff scheduling can be a problem during holidays, off shifts, or following a dramatic increase in the census. The nurse who was communicating with the woman might have had more volume in her case load and responsibilities than was reasonable in order to collect and process all the information needed to adequately care for individuals.

Prevention Strategies

Ensure competence and ask questions. Leaders must ensure that the competence and quality of all staff members are continually assessed and improved. Nurses are expected to be oriented and trained to meet care recipient needs in a timely manner. For example, nurses must be familiar with the medications they administer and be well prepared to make critical decisions about medications and medication timing. Nurses who are not comfortable with their knowledge or skill should ask questions and request additional training. Nurses are responsible for requesting training that ensures their own competence.

According to the procedures established by the organization in the example included earlier, the nurse was responsible for identifying the presence of a problem in the test results (that is, a possible tumor) and bringing the study results to the physician's attention. Procedures for doing so include presenting all test results to the physician at a scheduled time of day so that he or she can review them and determine what action needs to be taken. Nurses who are knowledgeable about common negative and positive results can place results needing attention before the physician so that they are not accidentally overlooked. The physician is responsible for ensuring a call to the care recipient. Even if the study results are entirely negative, under normal operating procedure, the nursing staff should make the physician aware of the results. The physician would then direct the office staff or nurse to call the care recipient.

Inform supervisor of unsafe staffing situations. Leaders need to ensure that nurses are able to

care for individuals in a timely and effective manner. With the previous example in mind, this means having time to evaluate the laboratory and X-ray results received in the office. In this scenario, a lack of sufficient staffing may have hindered the nurse's ability to take the time to sufficiently notify the physician of test results. Scheduling time for nurses' review of laboratory and radiographic results is critical. This can be performed at the end of the day to assure receipt of the maximum number of test results. If results are pending for tests that were performed or ordered that day, there should be a procedure to hold the record out of file for follow up at a subsequent time. If the record is filed away at the end of the work day, a tickler system can alert the office staff that test results are pending and that they need to be followed up on if not received within a set period of time. For example, mammograms may be read only on Tuesdays and Thursdays in some smaller organizations, although they could be performed daily. The office staff needs to know when a reasonable time frame for receipt of test results has been exhausted and when follow-up is required. Processes should be designed to minimize variation, which increases the likelihood of error.

Root Cause 3: Inadequate Assessment

Sentinel Event Example: Incomplete Assessment.

An 87-year old woman with urosepsis enters an emergency department (ED) at 8:00 AM and is evaluated by an ED nurse. The woman is frail, diaphoretic, and has a fever of 102.6° Fahrenheit. She is admitted to the hospital. The nurse places the woman's record in the box outside the woman's room, indicating a priority designation in order to call the ED physician's attention to the woman's condition. Anticipating the need for intravenous therapy, the nurse starts a peripheral line.

Approximately 15 minutes later, the ED physician comes into the room, reviews the record briefly, and determines that this woman may be septic. When contemplating antibiotic treatment for urosepsis in an elderly person, it is appropriate to order renal function tests and to await the results before administering antibiotics. The physician confirms the need for an IV line and orders renal function tests and a chest X-ray. There is a delay in the renal function testing. There also is a delay in the nursing and medical staff's initial assessment of the woman. An hour and a half elapses before the woman receives a physical examination by the ED physician at approximately 11:00 AM.

Two hours after she entered the ED, the woman's renal function tests have not been completed. The ED physician orders intravenous antibiotics to be given every six hours, pending the test results, and refers the woman to her attending physician for admission. The nurse in the emergency department makes the necessary arrangements to admit the woman. Another hour elapses before the woman is admitted to the 40-bed medical-surgical unit. The woman is received by a nurse on that unit and placed in a bed. Meanwhile, her renal test results are received, indicating a need for antibiotic therapy. The orders for IV antibiotics sit in the ED for an hour before they are transcribed and the pharmacy receives the order. Pharmacy staff deliver the antibiotics and place them in the medication room, noting the administration times of 10:00 AM, 4:00 PM, 10:00 PM, 4:00 AM.

The woman's vital signs are taken at 2:00 PM, at which point, she has been in the care setting for six hours. Her temperature has increased and is now 103.2° Fahrenheit. The nurse administers acetaminophen per order of the house officer. When the nurse comes into the room with the first dose of the woman's antibiotics at 3:45 PM, the woman is comatose and unresponsive. In septic shock, she is promptly transferred to the intensive care unit where she dies twelve hours later after having received only one dose of antibiotics.

This example illustrates the interaction of numerous root causes that contributed to a sentinel event, including inadequate communication, lack of information availability, inadequate continuity of care, and inadequate assessment, the latter of which is addressed in this section. Emergency departments are very busy places in many communities and often, the adequacy of staffing is an issue. Delays in treatment constitute a serious problem in such an environment. The medical and nursing staff should have assessed the woman promptly and reassessed her in order to track her increased fever. Assessments must be completed within the time frame specified by organization policy. Thorough assessment helps to ensure proper treatment. The woman in this example should

have received antibiotics as soon as there was a reasonable certainty that she was septic or had the potential to become septic. The orders for antibiotics should have been clearly written for immediate administration. This lacking, the woman went to the medical-surgical unit where the routine protocol for medication administration was followed.

Each discipline is responsible for recommending the number of staff necessary to complete assessments in a timely fashion. Leaders are responsible for ensuring safe staffing levels that ensures care timeliness. This is critical. For example, delay in recognition of a laboring mother's prolapsed cord in a busy labor and delivery suite could mean the difference between life and death for a fetus in delivery. Monitoring the fetus' heart rate ensures that the mother's contractions are productive and not destructive to the fetus. The nursing staff specifically must assess a prolapsed cord by digital examination. In some health care organizations, nurses are not trained to conduct such examinations. The result could be a serious delay in the diagnosis of a prolapsed cord.

Prevention Strategies

Perform initial nursing assessment within the time frame specified by organization policy. Prompt assessment helps to ensure prompt diagnosis and treatment in all care settings. Emergency departments present particular challenges to timeliness. In the example above, it is likely that the emergency department nurse was following a policy that treatment is not conducted in the emergency room, but relegated to nursing staff in medical-surgical units. Nurse and physician leaders must address this policy. Because there are limited nursing personnel in many emergency departments, moving patients through the emergency department and out into care units becomes imperative. It may not be entirely clear that a dose of antibiotics could save a life, but it has been well established that urinary tract infections and pneumonia in elderly, compromised individuals can lead to septicemia and serious failure of body systems in a relatively short period of time. The nurse's role is pivotal in assuring the necessary care in a timely fashion.

Ensure staffing and training necessary to perform assessments in a timely fashion. Staffing adequacy and timely assessments go hand-in-hand. In the scenario of the prolapsed cord, the nurse supervisor should analyze the need for and availability of staff in the labor and delivery suite who are trained to conduct definitive assessments. At the very least, the nurse needs to have available the personnel (attending or resident obstetrical staff) or be trained in recognizing and evaluating fetal heartbeat decelerations. Obstetrical residents and interns in teaching hospitals can perform a digital examination to assess the position of the baby and the potential for a prolapsed cord. The nurse in a community hospital where there are fewer deliveries needs to be trained at a different level. He or she needs to have the skills to provide even more in-depth assessment, including digital examination. The nurse also needs the skill and competence to address a prolapsed cord event when it does occur.

Reassess regularly to monitor care interventions. Appropriate nursing care involves regularly reassessing the care recipient's response to care. Delays in reassessing or monitoring the individual can lead to adverse occurrences. For example, continuously monitoring a woman in labor in the delivery suite is imperative. As the stages of labor progress and delivery comes closer, the potential for difficulty increases. The required nurse-to-patient ratio changes as the woman progresses through labor. Problems can arise, especially with women who have not had sufficient prenatal care and hence may have latent problems that are not evident or anticipated earlier. The physician must be summoned at just the right time as labor progresses. In organizations where there is no house staff, the nurse will need to make that decision independently.

Usually, criteria have been developed to allow for a consistent decision mechanism for the nurse. Modern monitoring techniques allow the nurse to monitor care recipients from a centralized location. These monitors are equipped with alarms that must be responded to promptly. For example, if it becomes evident that the fetal heartbeat is slowing, the nurse must assure a prompt response. Many smaller community hospitals do not have central moni-

toring. This makes it imperative for the nursing staff to frequently review the tracing to assess for decelerations in fetal heart rate.

Inadequate monitoring and reassessment contributed to the sentinel event described previously for the 87-year-old woman with urosepsis. With severely compromised individuals, the nursing staff must recognize the signs of decompensation and increasing illness. Nurses must evaluate the individual's present condition, compare it to the past reported condition, and apply principles of critical thinking and deductive reasoning to determine care needs. Nurses' ability to identify that an individual's condition is getting worse can be critical to the person's survival.

Communicate all changes thoroughly and quickly. Experience, skill, presence of mind, and ability to communicate effectively are all good attributes for nurses and all other health care team members. A delay in the communication of a prolapsed cord, for example, could result in a fetus' death. If the life-threatening situation to the fetus cannot be alleviated with first-hand intervention, then a cesarean section must occur. The nurse will need to summon support while acting to alleviate the pressure on the umbilical cord. Mechanisms to summon assistance are critical. Colleagues either take over portions of the individual's care while the nurse works with telephone operators to get the physician into the hospital immediately or communicates what is transpiring to a colleague or clerical person who can then make the necessary phone calls. Staff will need to rally together to assure quick results for the laboring woman while still attending to the needs of other individuals in the labor suite. The quick recruitment of the nursing supervisor to assist with calling the anesthesiologist in anticipation of a cesarean section is an example of a team working together and communicating well.

Root Cause 4: Inadequate Information Management

Sentinel Event Example: Mismanagement of Information. *A 75-year-old man who had triple vessel bypass surgery a month ago is accepted for home care by a visiting nurses association (VNA). The local medical center's discharge-planning department*

reports that the man's care will be quite involved. He is a diabetic who does not comply with dietary recommendations. He has only marginal circulation in his lower extremities, is a risk for stroke, and is on a host of medications that will require close monitoring. The man's wife is disabled and cannot contribute to her husband's care or oversight.

The man's medications include Warfarin, a drug used to thin the blood and decrease the likelihood of clot formation, and Tegretol, a drug used in some instances as a mild analgesic with specific neurological advantages for trigeminal neuralgia. These two drugs interact to increase (potentiate) anticoagulation. International Normalized Ratio (INR) is one of the tests used to indicate blood clotting ability. A normal INR is 1. The decreased clotting factor that generally is desired is between 2 to 3, meaning that it takes blood about twice the time to clot in an adequately treated patient. Regulation of medication doses is critical. An INR of 4 to 7 could lead to bleeding that could go beyond superficial bruising and actually affect vital organs including brain, bowel, heart, and so forth.

The VNA receives a copy of the man's discharge summary and a copy of the interagency referral form. The information is limited. The VNA also receives the name of a primary care physician who has been assigned to the man's care and has only seen him once while in the hospital. After the first visit to the man's home, the nurse reviews the medications and helps him organize a pill dispenser so that he knows what to take in the morning, mid day, and at night for seven days. The VNA nurse will visit the man on Tuesdays, Thursdays, and Saturdays. On the Tuesday of the second week, the nurse draws blood samples and delivers them to the laboratory. The physician's office receives the results showing an INR of 5.5. The physician files the results and does not act on them.

A week goes by and the visiting nurse, having complied with his responsibility, does not check with the physician's office for the laboratory results, assuming that they were probably in order. If there had been a problem, the nurse reasons that the physician would have phoned new orders to the pharmacy and notified him. On Thursday, the nurse goes to the man's home and finds no one there. The man had been admitted to the hospital after collapsing at home the night before. He travels to the hospital and locates the man's wife in the ICU waiting room surrounded by dis-

traught family. The man is on a ventilator in the ICU, fully obtunded, and in a vegetative state. He suffered a stroke. The nurse manager of the ICU informs the VNA nurse that the man's bleed was due to a significantly elevated Prothrombin time, with an INR of 7.0.

Clearly, the attending physician had a responsibility to contact the visiting nurse with the results of the INR. However, the nurse had equal responsibility to follow up non-forthcoming results with a call to the physician's office. For a care recipient such as the man described in this example, vigilance and oversight are very important. The man did not have enough information to question the results, and his wife was not able to help in managing his treatment. The man required education on the association of Tegretol and Warfarin and the probability of their potentiating effects. The delayed review of pending results and the failure to address information critical to the man's care compromised the care provided, resulting in a fatal bleed.

The transmission of data and information must be timely and accurate. In addition, the information must be acted upon in order to meet care recipient needs. If information is not transmitted at a time of critical value, or managed and acted upon appropriately by health care professionals, treatment can be delayed. Treatment could also be delayed when

- information retrieval systems do not allow off-shift staff to access information;
- ambulatory and emergency information is not part of the retrieval system;
- information is not stored in a central location; and
- information is not tracked, and therefore the clinical record may not be present and its location unknown.

The care recipient's clinical record, logs that are kept on the unit, and computer screens that trigger the viewer to address pending test results are all information management systems that support the individual's care and help reduce the likelihood of treatment delays. If these systems fail to prompt an action on the part of the responsible caregiver, their efficacy has in some way been compromised.

Laboratory test results are communicated to care settings in a number of ways. Some organizations have a computerized system that notes the results on the record as soon as they are obtained in the laboratory. In some such circumstances, staff may miss noting critical values. Or, if the system requires the ordering physician to look up results from a terminal in the hospital, results may be missed entirely until some adverse event occurs. In many instances, laboratories will call care units if the critical values (sometimes called "panic" values) are grossly out of range. If for any reason the laboratory cannot reach a staff member on the nursing unit, or the laboratory technologist speaks with a staff member who forgets to communicate the value, the information may sit on the care recipient's record and be noted too late to be appropriately addressed.

Nurses must be part of the process of developing and implementing appropriate information and communication systems. How is information communicated regarding the fact that an individual's blood has been drawn for a test, for example? How does the nursing staff know when and what tests have been obtained, and what results are pending so that they can make decisions to safely alter care until results have been received? Is there a log at the nursing station that details which tests have been obtained, for example? What information systems can be improved to call critical aspects of care to the attention of the nursing staff when medication and laboratory values must be correlated?

The example above illustrates the critical importance of timely and thorough information management and, as discussed earlier, complete caregiver communication. When an individual does not follow dietary recommendations, fluctuations in clotting factor are exceedingly difficult to control. Nurses caring for this person must

- be knowledgeable about all the medications the individual is taking and the over the counter (OTC) preparations that he may also be using. Did the nurse conduct an adequate assessment of the medications that the man in the example was taking? Did she ascertain whether the man was using alter-

native therapies that might enhance the effects of one or another medication? Often care recipients listen to advertisements on television about supplements such as St. John's Wort and Ginco-Biloba and assume that they will feel better once they start taking these supplements. They often give no thought to the impact that the OTC supplements may have on the effect of prescription medications.

- know when the care recipient is to see his or her physician and when values will be drawn. Often visiting nurses are actually drawing the blood for the physician, but rarely see test results first.

- coordinate with the physician's office to understand when values need to be drawn and how to follow up with the physician's office on assisting the care recipient to alter medication doses, as necessary. The visiting nurse in this example could have contacted the physician's office to see what the results were and if they had followed up on the results and called in a change of dose of Warfarin. Failure in the system for communication of critical laboratory values in this instance was not entirely the responsibility of the home care agency. All test results must be followed up on and communication between care providers in the outpatient and home care setting is just as critical as in the inpatient setting.

- understand the individual's diet and monitor it on an ongoing basis. The man in this example will have received some of the do's and don'ts about Warfarin on discharge from the hospital. However, since dietary compliance has been an issue in the control of the man's diabetes and heart condition, it is likely that compliance would also be an issue with anti-coagulative therapy. Dietary and pharmacy staff can assist and reinforce drug–diet interactions during patient education.

Prevention Strategies

Document care provided and response to care. Timely completion of clinical records is critical to quality care and to the prevention of sentinel events related to treatment delays. Nurses must document the care they provide and the individual's response to care. The clinical record is an imperfect communication medium. However, documentation of care in the clinical record often is a key method used by caregivers to communicate information. Therefore, it is essential. If information is received and filed in the record without being addressed or acted upon by the appropriate individual, the information is as good as lost. In such cases, information management certainly has fallen short of expectations and the purposes for which the record was designed.

Act in a timely and appropriate manner on information received. Clinical records must be designed in a way that ensures that information that is filed in the record is seen and acted upon by the appropriate individual(s). This includes information about the results of tests. If the record shows that a test has been ordered and obtained, there must be a system to match the results with that order for the test. In all settings, nurses help to ensure that this happens. The nursing role is particularly important in settings, such as home care, without several layers of providers who might have need for the results.

In the home care setting, the nurse often is the only professional who has a need for that information. A home care nurse's documentation acts as a reminder and as a trigger or tickler for another nurse who may be substituting during vacations, days off, or times of emergency. Records should include a section that addresses pending results. When home care providers perform tests on individuals, the results will, most likely, go to the ordering physician. The laboratory performing the test should either place a flag on the report to the physician's office suggesting a follow-up with the visiting nurse, or the laboratory should be encouraged to send a copy of the test results to the home care agency for inclusion in their files.

Ensure availability of the clinical record. Clinical records must be available to all those requiring the information in order to provide safe and timely care. If a home care agency, for example, allows a nurse to keep his or her records with him or her in the field, the nurse's car essentially becomes the record room. In such cases,

clerical staff in the home office is not able to file information and will need to go through assignment records to determine the nurse providing care to each individual. Under such situations, a report of a test, or an order from a physician, or other important information may be held in a box for the nurse who may only go through the material once or twice a week and file the material in the care recipient's record. Some home care agencies have devised systems of duplicate records—those that can accompany the nurse and those that stay in the office. In these cases, a system should be in place to assure that the two records contain the identical information. Many organizations are considering or implementing electronic record systems, which help ensure the availability of up to date clinical records and can permit access from multiple locations.

Other information management issues as they relate to physician's offices and patient care units in hospitals have been addressed earlier.

Root Cause 5: Environment of Care

Sentinel Event Example: Faulty Equipment. *Staff in an organization decide to centralize telemetry in a single location. The number of individuals on telemetry has increased sharply in the organization, up from an average of only 20 individuals, about four years ago. This results from the lack of criteria for triaging individuals off telemetry. Hence, physicians leave their patients on telemetry for entire hospital stays. However, increased telemetry capability has had a positive effect on moving individuals through the intensive care unit.*

The telemetry equipment, which is about 15 years old, is located in a fourth-floor room. Two staff members watch the monitors for as many as 126 care recipients located throughout the hospital. Yellow "post-it" notes taped to the side of each monitor indicate the care recipient's name and room number. Unit telephone numbers where the individuals are receiving care appear on a large board behind the monitor watchers.

Unbeknownst to the monitor watchers, the alarms for several of the oldest monitors are not operating properly. Additionally, the monitor watchers have disabled the alarms on some of the older equipment because their constant sounding in reaction to artifact is dis-

tracting and annoying. The monitor watchers feel comfortable that the critical alarms will sound if there is a lethal arrhythmia.

An individual on telemetry on one of the old monitors that is not operating properly develops life threatening arrhythmia at 1:30 AM. Due to the equipment's inoperative alarm system, the monitor watcher does not notice the arrhythmia for 25 to 30 minutes. At that point, the watcher determines that something must be awry with the equipment. She calls the individual's unit to notify the nurse to assess the care recipient. The phone rings and rings because the two nurses and one aide are attending to other care recipients and away from the desk.

Sensing a protracted delay, and not aware of how long the care recipient has been in ventricular tachycardia, the monitor watcher calls a code for the individual's room. The code team arrives and finds the nursing staff trying to respond to a code that they were not aware of on the unit. Resuscitation is initiated but is not successful. Death is deemed to be the result of missed detection of a fatal arrhythmia due to equipment failure.

In this scenario, even following appropriate policies and procedures could have serious and deadly effect. Care recipients are on telemetry due to problems with their heart rates and rhythms. Equipment failures, resulting in treatment delays, can lead to death or serious injury. Old equipment that frequently experiences false alarms is dangerous. Newer systems for telemetry that notify the responsible nurse via a pager may be appropriate, but all systems must be tested and maintained as per manufacturers' guidelines and organization policy.

Prevention Strategies

Help ensure proper safety and maintenance of equipment. Equipment function is paramount to the timely provision of safe care. Nurses need to know that the technology being used to monitor, to deliver drugs to, or to ventilate individuals in their care (among other functions), is in optimal functioning order. Nurses should not take for granted proper compliance with equipment maintenance. They can help identify faulty or improperly maintained equipment that might lead to a treatment delay and

resulting sentinel event. They need to know who is responsible for preventive maintenance and repair. Nurses may be so busy, for example, that when they identify a piece of equipment that is malfunctioning, they may exchange it for another that is functioning appropriately. They may accidentally place the broken piece of equipment in a dirty utility room, where the next unsuspecting nurse uses it on a care recipient with devastating effect. Nurses need to be aware of and follow organization policy and procedures and quarantine faulty equipment for maintenance, regardless of the time of day.

Participate on teams evaluating the purchase of new equipment. Nurses can help to identify new equipment that will reduce the likelihood of sentinel events.

Use equipment safely. Leaders need to ensure that nurses receive effective and adequate education on proper equipment use. Leaders in the example above should have been aware that remote monitoring using the old monitors introduced new risks and could cause delays in notifying the caregiver that the patient was experiencing problems. Had the biomedical engineer run the appropriate tests of the old telemetry equipment following its installation in the new monitor room on the fourth floor, he or she might have seen that the alarms on some of the old machines were not correctly hooked up and suggested that the project be scrapped or that the old monitors not be used until such time as repairs and adjustments could be made.

Advocate for system backup. Wherever equipment, new or old, is part of care and treatment, the design and implementation of redundant systems can help to ensure care recipient safety. If a ventilator or monitor fails, an individual should not have to die. The nurse should be able to implement interim measures to sustain the person until a new ventilator is secured. If a telemetry monitor fails, the nurse should have easily at his or her disposal the systems to evaluate the care recipient's rhythm until the equipment is back in optimal working order. Staff must recognize and plan for equipment limitations.

Closing Comment

In each phase of care, many opportunities exist for systems to break down, leading to delays in treatment. Delays in testing and obtaining test results, delays in implementing care guidelines, delays with the performance and documentation of history, physicals, and assessments, and delays in replacing or repairing faulty equipment can corrupt the process of establishing care priorities based on identified needs. These delays can lead to unexpected and adverse consequences. As critical health care team members, nurses are well-positioned to help reduce the likelihood of untoward events resulting from treatment delays.

Chapter 10:

Concluding Comments

The preceding nine chapters provided proactive strategies nurses can use to help prevent sentinel events in all types of health care organizations. Nurses can help prevent sentinel events, but they certainly are not responsible for the whole task of preventing sentinel events organizationwide. Nursing is a critical but single discipline represented on multidisciplinary health care teams. The whole team must be working to prevent sentinel events. So must the systems and processes established by organization leaders. As mentioned earlier, faulty systems and processes cause sentinel events, *not* individuals.

In the next few decades, nurses will continue to play a major role in planning and driving change to achieve improved safety, improved care, and improved outcomes for health care recipients. Their active leadership and participation in system design and redesign efforts will make a difference. So will their ability to identify and report hazardous conditions, close calls or near misses, and sentinel events so that all staff can learn from mistakes and improve performance and safety. Nurses must be involved from the unit level through the national level in the development of safe health care systems and processes.

The next several decades will also bring continued advances in technology and medicine. As a result, nurses increasingly will be called upon "to fill roles that will require increased professional judgment, supervision and direction of work of others, management of complex systems that span the traditional boundaries of service settings, and clinical autonomy," notes one IOM report.[1] Ongoing education, training, and competence assessment for nurses must focus,

among other areas, on new technology, interdisciplinary team care, care management, and new modes of care delivery.

"Clearly, a strong education base will be required to provide (nurses) with the needed preparation for their expected future roles in various settings," says an IOM committee.[1] Recommendations from experts about approaches to ensure nurse competence, such as re-licensure and certification, abound in the literature. A survey recently released by the American Nurses Credentialing Center indicates that a statistically significant portion of surveyed certified registered nurses reported that the continuing education required of certification enhanced their ability to identify potential errors and intervene proactively, thereby reducing the incidence of health care error.[2] The IOM advocates for periodic re-examinations and re-licensing by health professional licensing bodies of doctors, nurses, and other key providers on both competence and knowledge of safety practices.[3]

Whatever approach is used, ongoing nursing competence must be assured. Joint Commission standards and the ANA's *Code for Nurses* are clear on the need to maintain competence. The safety of individuals depends upon leaders, nurses, and other health care team members doing their part to attain and maintain competence, communicate appropriately and thoroughly, and work as an integrated collaborative team. Individuals receiving care in health care organizations must receive safe care. As frontline advocates for care recipients, nurses are well-positioned to help improve health care safety organizationwide and nationwide.

References

1. Wunderlich GD, Sloan FA, Davis CK: *Nursing Staff in Hospitals and Nursing Homes: Is It Adequate?* Report from the Institute of Medicine's Committee on the Adequacy of Nurse Staffing in Hospitals and Nursing Homes. Washington, DC: National Academy Press, 1996, p 87.

2. Foley M: Written testimony of the American Nurses Association before the Senate Committee on Health, Education, Labor and Pensions on Medical Errors, Jan 26, 2000. Web site: *www.nursingworld.org/gova/federal/legis/testimon/ 2000/mf0126htm.*

3. Institute of Medicine report: *To Err Is Human: Building a Safer Health System.* Washington, DC: National Academy Press, 2000, p 12.

Selected Resources

Joint Commission Publications
Newsletters

Sentinel Event Alert

- Blood transfusion errors: Preventing future occurrences. Issue 10, Aug 30, 1999.
- Fatal falls: Lessons for the future. Issue 14, Jul 12, 2000.
- High-alert medications and patient safety. Issue 11, Nov 19, 1999.
- Infant abductions: Preventing future occurrences. Issue 9, Apr 9, 1999.
- Infusion pumps: Preventing future adverse events. Issue 15, Nov 30, 2000.
- Inpatient suicides: Recommendations for prevention. Issue 7, Nov 6, 1998.
- Kernicterus threatens healthy newborns. Issue 18, Apr 2001.
- Lessons learned: Fires in the home care setting. Issue 17, Mar 20, 2001.
- Lessons learned: Wrong-site surgery. Issue 6, Aug 28, 1998.
- Look-alike, sound-alike drug names. Issue 19, May 2001.
- Medication error prevention—Potassium chloride. Issue 1, Feb 27, 1998.
- Medicinal gas mix-ups. Issue 21, Jul 2001.
- Operative and postoperative complications: Lessons for the future. Issue 12, Feb 4, 2000.
- Preventing needlestick and sharps injuries. Issue 22, Aug 2001.
- Preventing restraint deaths. Issue 8, Nov 18, 1998.

Joint Commission Benchmark

- Asking the "suicide question": Assess thoroughly and often to reduce risk. 1(6):1–3, Aug 1999.
- Catch them before they fall with multidisciplinary care plans. 2(12):1–3, Dec 2000.
- Preventing patient falls: Keeping patients safe without restraint. 1(9):1–3, Nov 1999.
- Scan your horizon for clear sailing: Preventing sentinel events before they happen. 1(1):1–3, Mar 1999.

Monographs

Medication Use: A Systems Approach to Reducing Errors (1998)

Preventing Adverse Events in Behavioral Health Care: A Systems Approach to Sentinel Event (1999)

Preventing Medication Errors: Strategies for Pharmacist (2001)

Preventing Patient Suicide (2000)

Reducing Restraint Use in the Acute Care Environment (1998)

Root Cause Analysis in Health Care: Tools and Techniques (2000)

Sentinel Events: Evaluating Cause and Planning Improvement (1998)

Storing and Securing Medications (1998)

Using Hospital Standards to Prevent Sentinel Events (2001)

What Every Hospital Should Know About Sentinel Events (2000)

Other Articles/Publications

Agency for Healthcare Research and Quality: *Medical errors: The scope of the problem.* Fact Sheet, Publication No. AHRQ 00-PO37, Rockville, MD: Feb 2000.

Agency for Healthcare Research and Quality: *20 tips to help prevent medical errors.* Patient Fact Sheet, Publication No. 00-PO38, Rockville, MD: Feb 2000.

Aiken LH, Smith HL, Lake ET: Lower Medicare mortality among a set of hospitals known for good nursing care. *Medical Care* 32(8):771–787, 1994.

American Hospital Association (AHA): *Hospital Nurse Recruitment and Retention, A Source Book for Executive Management.* No date. Chicago: AHA.

American Nurses Association (ANA): *Code for Nurses with Interpretive Statements.* Washington, DC: ANA, 1985.

American Nurses Association (ANA): *Nurse Staffing and Patient Outcomes in the Inpatient Hospital Setting.* Washington, DC: ANA, 2000.

American Nurses Association (ANA): *Nursing Care Report Card for Acute Care.* Washington, DC: ANA, 1995.

American Nurses Association (ANA): *Nursing's Social Policy Statement.* Washington, DC: ANA, 1995.

American Nurses Association (ANA): *Standards of Clinical Nursing Practice: 2nd Edition.* Washington, DC: ANA, 1998.

American Organization of Nurse Executives (AONE): *Nurse recruitment and retention study.* Chicago: AONE, Jan 2000.

American Society of Anesthesiologists: Questions and answers about transfusion practices, 3rd edition. Park Ridge, IL, 1997.

American Society of Health-System Pharmacists: ASHP offers hospital and health-system CEO's practical recommendations for improving medication-use safety. ASHP Online: *www.ashp.org/public/news/breaking/hrm_memo.html.*

American Society of Health-System Pharmacists: Suggested definitions and relationships among medication misadventures, medication errors, adverse drug events, and adverse drug reactions, Jan 15, 1998. Web address: *www.ashp.com/ public/proad/mederror/draftdefin.html.*

American Society of Health-System Pharmacists: Survey of top patient concerns: Research report, September 1999. ASHP Online: *www.ashp.org/public/proad/hsp_week/cons_out.html.*

American Society of Health-System Pharmacists: Top-priority actions for preventing adverse drug events in hospitals: recommendations of an expert panel. *Am J Health-Syst Pharm* 53:747–51, 1996. In Bates DW, et al: Incidence of adverse drug events and potential adverse drug events. *JAMA* 274(1):29–34, 1995.

ANA Board of Directors: Position statements: Joint statement on maintaining professional and legal standards during a shortage of nursing personnel. Aug 1992. Web site: *www.nursing-world.org/readroom/position/joint/jtshort.htm.*

Appropriateness of Minimum Nurse Staffing Ratios in Nursing Homes. HCFA Report to Congress, Aug 1, 2000. Web site: *www.hcfa.gov/medicaid/ reports/rp700hmp.htm.*

Bates DW, et al: Incidence of adverse drug events and potential adverse drug events. *JAMA* 274(1):29–34, 1995.

Bates DW, et al: Effect of computerized physician order entry and a team intervention on prevention of serious medication errors. *JAMA* 280(15):1311–1316, 1998.

Bates DW, et al: Serious falls in hospitalized patients: Correlates and resource utilization. *Am J of Med* 99:137–143, Aug 1995.

Bates DW, et al: The impact of computerized physician order entry on medication error prevention. *J AM Med Inform Assoc* 6(4):313–321, 1999.

Berwick DM. Developing and testing changes in delivery of care. *Ann Intern Med.* 1998; 128: 651–656.

Beyers M (ed): *The Business of Nursing.* Chicago: American Hospital Publishing, 1996.

Bogner MS (ed): *Human Error in Medicine.* Hillsdale, NJ: Lawrence Erlbaum Associates, 1994.

Bongar BM (ed): *Risk Management with Suicidal Patients.* New York: Guilford Press, 1998.

Bootman JL, Harrison DL, Cox E: The health care costs of drug-related morbidity and mortality in nursing facilities. *Arch Intern Med* 1997;157:1531–1536.

Bowers DM: Closing the door on wanderers. *Journal of Healthcare Protection Management* 15(1):109–117, 1998/1999.

Brennan TA, et al: Identification of adverse events occurring during hospitalization. *Annals of Internal Medicine* 112(3):221–226,1990.

Brennan T, et al: Incidence of adverse events and negligence in hospitalized patients: Results of the Harvard Medical Practice Study I. *New England Journal of Medicine* 324:370–376, 1991.

Buerhaus P, Wakefield M: *Perspectives on the Nursing Shortage: A Blueprint for Action.* Chicago: American Hospital Association/American Organization of Nurse Executives, Nov 2000.

Cardell R, Horton-Deutsch: A model for assessment of inpatient suicide potential, *Arch of Psych Nursing* 8(6):366–372.

Cardell R, Quinnett P, Bratcher K: *QPRT-H Suicide Risk Management Inventory-Hospital Version.* Spokane, WA: Cardell, Quinnett, and Bratcher, 1999.

Cohen MR (ed): *Medication Errors.* Washington, DC: American Pharmaceutical Association, 1999.

Coleman IC: Medication errors: Picking up the pieces. *Drug Topics,* Mar 15, 1999, pp 83–92.

Conley D, Schultz AA, Selvin R: The challenge of predicting patients at risk for falling: Development of the Conley Scale. *MEDSURG Nursing* 8(6):348–354, Dec 1999.

Cousins DD (ed): *Medication Use: A Systems Approach to Reducing Errors.* Oakbrook Terrace, IL: Joint Commission, 1998.

Croteau RJ, Schyve PM: Proactively error-proofing health care processes. In Spath P (ed): *Error Reduction in Health Care.* San Francisco: Jossey-Bass Publishers, 2000, pp 179–198.

Dean BS, Barber ND: A validated, reliable method of scoring the severity of medication errors. *Am J Health-Syst Pharm* 56:57–62, 1999.

Despotis G: Current and evolving issues in transfusion therapy. Park Ridge, IL: American Society of Anesthesiologists 1999 Annual Refresher Course Lectures, No. 162.

Elliott SJ: Health care whistleblower legislation. *Health Law Alert,* Mar 2000. Milwaukee: vonBriesen, Purtell & Roper. Web site: *www.vonbriesen.com/whistleblower.htm.*

Escovitz A, Pathak DS, Schneider PJ (eds): *Improving the Quality of the Medication Use Process: Error Prevention and Reducing Adverse Drug Events.* Binghamton, NY: The Haworth Press, 1998.

Foley M: Written testimony of the American Nurses Association before the Senate Committee on Health, Education, Labor and Pensions on Medical Errors, Jan 26, 2000. Web site: *www.nursingworld.org/gova/federal/legis/ testimon/2000/mf0126htm.*

Gainey A: Caregiving: Focus on reducing restraints in SNFs. *Provider* 26(7):49–50, 2000.

Goodnough LT, et al: Transfusion medicine: Blood transfusion. *New England Journal of Medicine* 340:438–447, 1999.

Hackel R, Butt L, and Banister G: How nurses perceive medication errors. *Nursing Management* 27(1):31–34, 1996.

Harrington C, et al: Experts recommend minimum nurse staffing standards for nursing facilities in the United States. *The Gerontologist* 40(1):5–16, 2000.

Healthcare Risk Management: Confirm correct site, then apply your John Hancock, Mar 1999.

Hilfiker D: Facing our mistakes. *N Engl J Med* 310:118–122, Jan 12, 1984.

Howard-Ruben J: A new respect for pain. *Nursing Spectrum* 13(14):12–13, 2000.

Hudacek S: *Making a Difference—Stories from the Point of Care.* Indianapolis: Center Nursing Press, 2000.

Institute for Safe Medication Practices: A case riddled with latent and active failures. *ISMP Medication Safety Alert!* Feb 11, 1998. Web site: *www.ismp.org/MSAarticles/Latent.html.*

Institute for Safe Medication Practices: Evidence builds: Lack of focus on human factors allows error-prone devices. *ISMP Medication Safety Alert!* Jul 28, 1999. Web site: *www.ismp.org/MSAarticles/humanfactors.html.*

Institute for Safe Medication Practices: Lessons from Denver: Look beyond blaming individuals for errors. *ISMP Medication Safety Alert!* Feb 11, 1998. Web site: *www.ismp.org/MSAarticles/Denver.html.*

Institute for Safe Medication Practices: Maintaining patient safety in the face of staff reduction. *ISMP Medication Safety Alert,* Oct 20, 1999. Web site: *www.ismp.org/MSAarticles/staffing.html.*

Institute for Safe Medication Practices: The "five rights." *ISMP Medication Safety Alert,* Apr 7, 1999. Web site: *www.ismp.org/MSAarticles/fiverights.html.*

Institute of Medicine Report: *To Err is Human: Building a Safer Health System.* Washington, DC: National Academy Press, 2000.

Institute of Medicine report: *Crossing the Quality Chasm: A New Health System for the 21st Century.* Washington, DC: National Academy Press, 2001.

Jacobs DG (Ed): *The Harvard Medical School Guide to Suicide Assessment and Intervention.* San Francisco: Josssey-Bass, 1999.

Kaiser Family Foundation and the Agency for Healthcare Research and Quality: *National Survey on Americans as Health Care Consumers: An Update on the Role of Quality Information.* Dec 2000. Web site: *www.kff.org.*

Knauf RA, et al: *Implementing Nursing's Report Card: A Study of RN Staffing, Length of Stay and Patient Outcomes.* Washington, DC: American Nurses Association, 1997.

Knox GE, et al: Downsizing, reengineering and patient safety: Numbers, new-ness and resultant risk. *J Health Risk Manag* 1999; 19:18–25.

Leape LL: Address to National Patient Safety Foundation news conference, Chicago, Oct 7, 1997.

Leape LL: Error in medicine. *JAMA* 272(23): 1851–1857, 1994.

Leape LL: Reducing adverse drug events: Lessons from a breakthrough series collaborative. *Jt Comm J on Qual Improve,* forthcoming publication.

Leape LL, et al: The nature of adverse events in hospitalized patients: Results of the Harvard Medical Practice Study. *New England Journal of Medicine* 324:377–384, 1991.

Leape LL, et al: Systems analysis of adverse drug events. *JAMA* 274 (1):35–43, 1995.

Leape LL, Berwick DM: Safe health care: Are we up to it? *BMJ* 320:725–726, 18 Mar 2000.

Linden JV, et al: Decrease in frequency of transfusion fatalities. *Transfusion* 37:243–244, 1997.

Linden JV, Kaplan HS: Transfusion errors: Causes and effects. *Transfusion Medicine Reviews* 8:169–183, 1994.

Manasse HR: Toward defining and applying a higher standard of quality for medication use in the United States. ASHP Online: *www.ashp.com/public/proad/mederror/pman.html,* 1999.

National Coordinating Council for Medication Error Reporting and Prevention: *NCC MERP taxonomy of medication errors.* Rockville, MD: U.S. Pharmacopeia, 1998.

National Patient Safety Foundation at the American Medical Association: *Public Opinion of Patient Safety Issues: Research Findings.* Sep 1997. Web site: *www.npsf.org.*

O'Leary DS: Editorial: Accreditation's role in reducing medical errors. *BMJ* 320:727–728, Mar 2000.

O'Leary D: Statement of the Joint Commission on Accreditation of Healthcare Organizations before the Committee on Health, Education, Labor and Pensions, U.S. Senate and the Subcommittee on Labor, Health and Human Services, and Education of the Senate Committee on Appropriations, Feb 22, 2000. Web site: *www.jcaho.org/govt/oleary_022200.html.*

Opus Communications: First Do No Harm: *A Practical Guide to Medication Safety and JCAHO Compliance.* Marblehead, MA: Opus Communications, Inc., 1999.

Patient fears persist. *Healthcare Business,* Jan/Feb 2000.

Pear R: U.S. health officials reject plan to report medical mistakes. *New York Times,* Jan 24, 2000, p 14A.

Pepper GA: Errors in drug administration by nurses. *Am J Health-Syst Pharm* 52:390–395, 1995.

Platts WE: Psychiatric patients: Premises liability and predicting patient elopement. *Journal of Healthcare Protection Management* 14(2):66–77, 1998.

Quality Interagency Coordination Task Force: *Doing what counts for patient safety: Federal actions to reduce medical errors and their impact.* Report to the President, Feb 2000.

Rabun JB: *For Healthcare Professionals: Guidelines on Prevention of and Response to Infant Abductions– Sixth Edition.* Arlington, VA: National Center for Missing & Exploited Children, Mar 2000.

Raschke RA, et al: A computer alert system to prevent injury from adverse drug events. *JAMA* 280(15):1317–1320, 1998.

Reason J: *Human Error.* Cambridge University Press, 1990.

Reason J: Human error: Models and management. *BMJ* 320:768–770, 18 Mar 2000.

Reason JT: *Managing the Risks of Organizational Accidents.* Aldershot, UK: Ashgate, 1997.

Rich D: Ask the Joint Commission: Automated dispensing devices. *Hosp Pharm,* Jun 2000.

Romig CL: Health policy issues: Developing a nurse-to-patient ratio policy. *AORN Journal,* Nov 2000. Web site: *www.aorn.org/journal/nov2khpi.htm.*

Schyve PM: Statement of the Joint Commission on Accreditation of Healthcare Organizations at the National Summit of Medical Errors and Patient Safety Research. Sep 11, 2000. Web site: *www.jcaho.org/sentinel/se_summit.html.*

Sexton JB, Thomas EJ, Helreich RL: Error, stress, and teamwork in medicine and aviation: Cross sectional surveys. *BMJ* 320:745–749, 18 Mar 2000.

Sharpe VA: *Medical Harm: Historical, Conceptual, and Ethical Dimensions of Iatrogenic Illness.* Cambridge, MA: Cambridge University Press, 1998.

Shneidman ES, Farberow NL, Litman RL (eds): *The Psychology of Suicide: A Clinician's Guide to Evaluation and Treatment.* Northvale, NJ: J. Aronson, 1994.

Sigma Theta Tau International, Nursing Honor Society: Dickenson-Hazard responds to *Chicago Tribune* articles. Sep 15, 2000. Web site: *www.nursingsociety.org.*

Spencer FC: Human error in hospitals and industrial accidents: Current concepts. *J Am College of Surgeons* 191(4):410–418, Oct 2000.

Spetz J: Hospital use of nursing personnel hold-ing steady through the 1990s. *JONA* 30(7/8): 344–346, Jul/Aug 2000.

Thomas E, et al: Incidence and types of adverse events and negligent care in Utah and Colorado. *Medical Care* 38:261–271, 2000.

Tissot E, et al: Medication errors at the administration stage in an intensive care unit. *Intensive Care Medicine* 25:353–359, 1999.

Trossman S: ANA, MNA support Dana-Farber nurses facing disciplinary action. *MassNurs News,* Apr/May 1999. Web site: *www.massnurses.org.*

When medicine hurts instead of helps: Preventing medication problems in older persons. Washington, DC: Alliance for Aging Research; 1998:1–12.

Wilson AL, et al: Computerized medication administration records decrease medication occurrences. *Pharm Pract Manager Q* 17(1):17–29, 1997.

Wunderlich GD, Sloan FA, Davis CK: *Nursing Staff in Hospitals and Nursing Homes: Is It Adequate?* Report from the Institute of Medicine's Committee on the Adequacy of Nurse Staffing in Hospitals and Nursing Homes. Washington, DC: National Academy Press, 1996.

Zarabozo C: Explosion in the medicine chest. *Health Care Finan Rev* 20(3):1–13, 1999.

Organizations

American Association of Suicidology
4201 Connecticut Avenue, NW
Suite 408
Washington, DC 20008
Phone: 202/237-2280
Fax: 202/237-2282
Web site: www.suicideology.org

American Foundation for Suicide Prevention
120 Wall Street, 22nd Floor
New York, NY 10005
Phone: 888/333-AFSP
Fax: 212/363-6237
Web site: www.afsp.org

American Pharmaceutical Association
2215 Constitution Avenue, N.W.
Washington, DC 20037
202/628-4410
Web site: www.aphanet.org

American Society of Health-System Pharmacists
7272 Wisconsin Avenue
Bethesda, MD 20814
301/657-3000
Web site: www.ashp.com

Center for Proper Medication Use
P.O. Box 13329
Philadelphia, PA 19101
215/895-1131
Web site: www.cpmu.org

Food and Drug Administration
Web site: www.fda.gov

Institute for Healthcare Improvement
135 Francis Street
Boston, MA 02215
617/754-4800
Web site: www.ihi.org

Institute for Safe Medication Practices
1800 Byberry Road, Suite 810
Huntington Valley, PA 19006
215/947-7797
Web site: www.ismp.org

National Association for Healthcare Quality
4700 W. Lake Avenue
Glenview, IL 60025
800/966-9392
Web site: www.nahq.org

Joint Commission on Accreditation of Healthcare Organizations
One Renaissance Boulevard
Oakbrook Terrace, IL 60181
630/792-5000
Web site: www.jcaho.org

Joint Commission Resources
One Renaissance Boulevard
Oakbrook Terrace, IL 60181
630/792-5000
Web site: www.jcrinc.com

The National Alliance for the Mentally Ill
200 North Glebe Road, Suite 1015
Arlington, VA 22203-3754
Phone: 800/950-6264
Fax: 703/524-9094
Web site: www.nami.org

National Coordinating Council for Medication Error Reporting and Prevention
Web site: www.nccmerp.org

National Depressive & Manic-Depressive
Association
730 N. Franklin Street, Suite 501
Chicago, IL 60610-3526
Phone: 800/826-3632
Fax: 312/642-7243
Web site: www.ndmda.org

National Institute of Mental Health
National Institutes of Health
NIMH Suicide Research Consortium
6001 Executive Boulevard, Room 8184,
MSC 9663
Bethesda, MD 20892-9663
Phone: 301/443-4513
Fax: 301/443-4279
Web site: www.nimh.nih.gov

National Mental Health Association
1021 Prince Street
Alexandria, VA 22314-2971
Phone: 800/969-NMHA
Fax: 703/684-5968
Web site: www.nmha.org

National Patient Safety Foundation
515 N. State Street
Chicago, IL 60610
312/464-4848
Web site: www.npsf.org

SA/VE-Suicide Awareness/Voices of Education
Box 24507
Minneapolis, MN 55424-0507
612/946-7998
Web Site: www.save.org

Suicide Information and Education Centre
#201, 1615-10th Avenue SW
Calgary, Alberta Canada T3C 0J7
Phone: 403/245-3900
Fax: 403/245-0299
Web site: www.siec.ca

Suicide Prevention Advocacy Network
5034 Odin's Way
Marietta, GA 30068
Phone: 888/649-1366
Fax: 770/642-1419
Web site: www.spanusa.org
E-mail: spanusa@mindspring.com

United States Pharmacopeia
12601 Twinbrook Parkway
Rockville, MD 20852
301/816-8216
Web site: www.usp.org

Appendix:

Safety and Health Care Error Reduction Standards

These standards are from the *2001 Comprehensive Accreditation Manual for Hospitals,* Update 1.

Patient Rights and Organization Ethics (RI)

Standard

RI.1.2.2   Patients and, when appropriate, their families are informed about the outcomes of care, including unanticipated outcomes.

Intent of RI.1.2.2

The responsible licensed independent practitioner or his or her designee clearly explains the outcome of any treatments or procedures to the patient and, when appropriate, the family, whenever those outcomes differ significantly from the anticipated outcomes.

Scoring for RI.1.2.2

Has the responsible licensed independent practitioner or his/her designee informed the patient and, when appropriate, the family, about the outcomes of care, including unanticipated outcomes?

Score 1   Always

Score 2   Usually

Score 3   Sometimes

Score 4   Rarely

Score 5   Never

1 2 3 4 5 NA

Education (PF)

Standard

PF.3.7   Education includes information about patient responsibilities in the patient's care.

Intent of PF.3.7

The safety of health care delivery is enhanced by the involvement of the patient, as appropriate to his/her condition, as a partner in the health care process. In addition, hospitals are entitled to reasonable and responsible behavior on the part of the patients and their families. The hospital identifies patient and family responsibilities and educates the patient and family about these responsibilities. Specific attention is directed at educating patients and families about their role in helping to facilitate the safe delivery of care.

Responsibilities include at least the following:

- **Providing information.** The patient is responsible for providing, to the best of his or her knowledge, accurate and complete information about present complaints, past illnesses, hospitalizations, medications, and other matters relating to his or her health. The patient and family are responsible for reporting perceived risks in their care and unexpected changes in the patient's condition. The patient and family help the hospital improve its understanding of the patient's environment by providing feedback about service needs and expectations.
- **Asking questions.** Patients are responsible for asking questions when they do not understand what they have been told about their care or what they are expected to do.
- **Following instructions.** The patient and family are responsible for following the care, service, or treatment plan developed. They should express any concerns they have about their ability to follow and comply with the proposed care plan or course of treatment. Every effort is made to adapt the plan to the patient's specific needs and limitations. When such adaptations to the treatment plan are not recommended, the patient and family are responsible for understanding the consequences of the treatment alternatives and not following the proposed course.
- **Accepting consequences.** The patient and family are responsible for the outcomes if they do not follow the care, service, or treatment plan.
- **Following rules and regulations.** The patient and family are responsible for following the hospital's rules and regulations concerning patient care and conduct.
- **Showing respect and consideration.** Patients and families are responsible for being considerate of the hospital's personnel and property.
- **Meeting financial commitments.** The patient and family are responsible for promptly meeting any financial obligation agreed to with the hospital.

Patients are educated about their responsibilities during the admission, registration, or intake process and as needed thereafter.

The patient's family or surrogate decision-maker assumes the above responsibility for the patient if the patient has been found by his or her physician to be incapable of understanding these responsibilities, has been judged incompetent in accordance with law, or exhibits a communication barrier.

The hospital informs each patient of his or her responsibilities either verbally, in writing, or both, based on hospital policy.

Patients are responsible for being considerate of other patients, helping control noise and disturbances, following smoking policies, and respecting others' property.

Continuum of Care (CC)

Standards

CC.4 The hospital ensures continuity over time among the phases of service to a patient.

CC.5 The hospital ensures coordination among the health professionals and services or settings involved in a patient's care.

Intent of CC.4 and CC.5

Care is coordinated throughout
- entry;
- assessment;
- diagnosis;
- planning;
- treatment; and
- transfer or discharge.

Throughout all phases, patient needs are matched with appropriate resources within the continuum (for example, special care units, skilled nursing facility, or community services). Transitions between levels of care are smooth. Coordination of services may involve promoting communication to facilitate family support, social work, nursing care, consultation or referral, primary physician care, or other follow-up. Communication and transfer of information between and among the health care professionals is essential to a seamless, safe, and effective process.

1 2 3 4 5 NA

Scoring for CC.4

Is there a process, which addresses the issues described in the intent, for transfer, referral, discontinuation of services, and discharge based on a patient's assessed needs?

Score 1   Always

Score 2   Usually

Score 3   Sometimes

Score 4   Rarely

Score 5   Never

1 2 3 4 5 NA

Scoring for CC.5

When a patient is accepted, referred, transferred, discharged or when services are discontinued, does the hospital use a process to receive appropriate information and to communicate appropriate information to subsequent care providers?

Score 1   Always

Score 2   Usually

Score 3   Sometimes

Score 4   Rarely

Score 5   Never

Improving Organization Performance (PI)

Standard

PI.2 New or modified processes are designed well.

Intent of PI.2

When processes, functions, or services are designed well, they draw on a variety of information sources. Good process design

a. is consistent with the organization's mission, vision, values, goals and objectives, and plans;

b. meets the needs of individuals served, staff, and others;

c. is clinically sound and current (for instance, use of practice guidelines, successful practices, information from relevant literature, and clinical standards);

d. is consistent with sound business practices;

e. incorporates available information from within the organization and from other organizations about potential risks to patients, including the occurrence of sentinel events* in order to minimize risks to patients affected by the new or redesigned process, function, or service;

f. includes analysis and/or pilot testing to determine whether the proposed design/redesign is an improvement; and

g. incorporates the results of performance-improvement activities.

The organization incorporates information related to these elements, when available and relevant, in the design or redesign of processes, functions, or services.

Scoring for PI.2

When available and relevant, do new or modified processes incorporate items a through g as described in the intent?

Score 1   Always

Score 2   Usually

Score 3   Sometimes

Score 4   Rarely

Score 5   Never

Standard

PI.3.1 The organization collects data to monitor its performance.

Intent of PI.3.1

Performance monitoring and improvement are data driven. The stability of important processes can provide the organization with information about its performance. Every organization must choose which processes and outcomes (and thus which types of data) are important to monitor based on its mission and the scope of care and services it provides. The leaders prioritize data collection based on the organization's mission, care and services provided, and populations served (see LD.4.2 for priority setting). Data that the organization considers for collection to monitor performance include the following:

- Performance measures related to accreditation and other requirements;
- Risk management;
- Utilization management;
- Quality control;
- Patient, family, and staff opinions, needs, perceptions of risks to patients, and suggestions for improving patient safety;
- Staff willingness to report medical/health care errors;
- Staff opinions and needs;
- Behavior management[†] procedures, if used;
- Outcomes of processes or services;
- Autopsy results, when performed;
- Performance measures from acceptable databases;
- Customer demographics and diagnoses;
- Financial data;
- Infection control surveillance and reporting;

---

* **sentinel event** A sentinel event is an unexpected occurrence involving death or serious physical or psychological injury, or risk thereof. Serious injury specifically includes loss of life or function. The phrase "or the risk thereof" includes any process variation for which a recurrence would carry a significant chance of a serious adverse outcome.

1 2 3 4 5 NA

[†] The use of basic learning techniques, such as biofeedback, reinforcement, or aversion therapy, to manage and improve an individual's behavior.

* To better measure the performance of organizations on how well they meet the needs, expectations, and concerns of individuals, the Joint Commission is moving from the term satisfaction toward the more inclusive term perception of care and service. By using this term, the organization will be prompted to assess not only individuals' and/or families' satisfaction with care or treatment, but also whether their needs and expectations are met by the organization.

1 2 3 4 5 NA

† **significant adverse drug reactions and significant medication errors** Unintended, undesirable, and unexpected effects of prescribed medications or medication errors that require discontinuing a medication or modifying the dose, require initial or prolonged hospitalization, result in disability, require treatment with a prescription medication, result in cognitive deterioration or impairment, are life threatening, result in death, or result in congenital anomalies.

‡ **Hazardous condition** Any set of circumstances (exclusive of the disease or condition for which the patient is being treated) which significantly increases the likelihood of a serious adverse outcome.

§ **root cause analysis** A process for identifying the basic or causal factor(s) that underlie variation in performance, including the occurrence or possible occurrence of a sentinel event.

- Research data;
- Performance data identified in various chapters of this manual; and
- The appropriateness and effectiveness of pain management.

Organizations are required to collect data about the needs, expectations, and satisfaction of individuals and organizations served. Individuals served and their family members can provide information that will give an organization insight about process design and functioning. The organization asks them about

- their specific needs and expectations;
- their perceptions* of how well the organization meets these needs and expectations;
- how the organization can improve; and
- how the organization can improve patient safety.

The organization can use a number of ways to get input from these groups, including satisfaction surveys, regularly scheduled meetings held with these groups, and focus groups.

Scoring for PI.3.1

a. Has the organization identified performance areas for which data will be collected?
b. Has the organization identified perception of care data for collection?
c. Has the organization identified patient safety data for collection?
d. Have the appropriate detail and frequency of data collection been determined?
e. Are data collected at the frequency and with the detail identified by the organization?

Score 1   a. through e.   Always

Score 2   a. through e.   Usually

Score 3   a. through e.   Sometimes

Score 4   a. through e.   Rarely

Score 5   a. through e.   Never

Standard

PI.4.3 Undesirable patterns or trends in performance and sentinel events are intensively analyzed.

Intent of PI.4.3

When the organization detects or suspects significant undesirable performance or variation, it initiates intense analysis to determine where best to focus changes for improvement. The organization initiates intense analysis when the comparisons show that

- levels of performance, patterns, or trends vary significantly and undesirably from those expected;
- performance varies significantly and undesirably from that of other organizations;
- performance varies significantly and undesirably from recognized standards; or
- when a sentinel event has occurred.

When monitoring performance of specific clinical processes, certain events always elicit intense analysis. Based on the scope of care or services provided, intense analysis is performed for the following:

- Confirmed transfusion reactions;
- Significant adverse drug reactions; and
- Significant medication errors and hazardous conditions.†‡

Intense analysis should also occur for those topics chosen by the leaders as performance-improvement priorities and priorities for proactive reduction in patient risk (see LD.1.4 and LD.5.2), or when undesirable variation occurs that changes the priorities. Intense analysis involves studying a process to learn in greater detail about how it is performed or how it operates, how it can malfunction, and how errors occur.

A root cause analysis§ is performed when a sentinel event occurs.

An intense analysis is also performed for the following:

- Major discrepancies, or patterns of discrepancies, between preoperative and postoperative (including pathologic) diagnoses, including those identified during the pathologic review of specimens removed during surgical or invasive procedures; and
- Significant adverse events associated with anesthesia use.

Standard

PI.4.4 The organization identifies changes that will lead to improved performance and improve patient safety.

Intent of PI.4.4

The organization uses the information from the data analysis to identify system changes that will improve performance or improve patient safety. Changes are identified based on the analysis of data from targeted study or from analysis of data from ongoing monitoring. A change is selected, and the organization plans to implement the change on a pilot test basis or across the organization. Performance measures are selected that help determine the effectiveness of the change and whether it resulted in an improvement (see PI.3.1.1, PI.3.1.2, and PI.3.1.3) once the change is implemented.

Scoring for PI.4.3

1 2 3 4 5 NA

a. Does the organization initiate intense analysis when comparisons indicate negative trends or that performance is significantly below the performance specifications?
b. Was a root cause analysis performed when a sentinel event occurred?
c. Is an intense analysis performed for all confirmed transfusion reactions?
d. Is an intense analysis performed for all significant adverse drug reactions?
e. Is an intense analysis performed for all significant medication errors and hazardous conditions?
f. Is an intense analysis performed for all major discrepancies between preoperative and postoperative diagnoses?
g. Is an intense analysis performed for adverse events or patterns of adverse events during anesthesia use?

Score 1   a. through g. Always (or not applicable to organization)

Score 2   a. Usually
               b. Usually

Score 3   a. Sometimes
               b. Sometimes

Score 4   a. Rarely
               b. Rarely

Score 5   a. through g. Never

Leadership (LD)

Standard

LD.1.4 The planning process provides for setting performance-improvement priorities and identifies how the hospital adjusts priorities in response to unusual or urgent events.

Intent of LD.1.4

The planning process provides the framework or criteria for establishing performance-improvement priorities. The planning process gives priority consideration to

- processes that affect a large percentage of patients;
- processes that place patients at risk if not performed well, if performed when not indicated, or if not performed when indicated; and
- processes that have been or are likely to be problem prone.

The hospital's priority setting is sensitive to emerging needs such as those identified through data collection and assessment, unanticipated adverse occurrences affecting patients, changing regulatory requirements, significant patient and staff needs, changes in the environment of care, or changes in the community.

Scoring for LD.1.4

1 2 3 4 5 NA

a. Does the planning process identify how priorities for performance improvement will be set?
b. Does the planning process identify how the hospital resets priorities in response to unusual or urgent events?

Score 1   a. Yes
               b. Yes

Score 5   a. No
               b. No

Standard

LD.1.8 The leaders and other relevant personnel collaborate in decision making.

Intent of LD.1.8

The hospital's leaders and directors of relevant departments collaborate in

- development of hospitalwide patient care programs, policies, and procedures that describe how patients' care needs are assessed and met;
- development and implementation of the hospital's plan for providing patient care;
- decision-making structures and processes;
- implementation of an effective and continuous program to measure, assess, and improve performance and improve patient safety.

1 2 3 4 5 NA

Scoring for LD.1.8

Do hospital leaders and other relevant personnel collaborate in the structures and processes related to

- development of hospitalwide patient care programs, policies, and procedures that describe how patients' care needs are assessed and met;
- development and implementation of the hospital's plan for providing patient care;
- decision-making structures and processes; and
- implementation of an effective and continuous program to measure, assess, and improve performance and improve patient safety?

Score 1   Yes

Score 3   Not consistently

Score 5   No

Standard

LD.3.2   The leaders foster communication and coordination among individuals and departments.

Intent of LD.3.2

To coordinate and integrate patient care and to improve patient safety, the leaders develop a culture that emphasizes cooperation and communication. An open communication system facilitates an interdisciplinary approach to providing patient care. The leaders develop methods for promoting communication among services, individual staff members, and less formal structures such as quality action teams, performance-improvement teams, or members of standing committees.

This leadership role is commonly referred to as coaching.

1 2 3 4 5 NA

Scoring for LD.3.2

Do hospital leaders foster systematic communication among departments and individuals?

Score 1   Yes

Score 3   Communication is not systematic.

Score 5   No

Standard

1 2 3 4 5 NA

LD.3.4.1   The leaders provide for mechanisms to measure, analyze, and manage variation in the performance of defined processes that affect patient safety.

Intent of LD.3.4.1

Inconsistency in the performance of processes, as intended by their design and described in organization policies and procedures, frequently leads to unanticipated and undesirable results. In order to minimize risk to patients due to such variation, the leaders ensure that the actual performance of processes identified as error-prone or high-risk regarding patient safety is measured and analyzed, and when significant variation is identified, appropriate corrective actions are taken to enhance the system(s).

At any given time, the performance of critical steps in at least one high-risk process is the subject of ongoing measurement and periodic analysis to determine the degree of variation from intended performance.

Scoring for LD.3.4.1

a. Do the leaders ensure that the actual performance of processes identified as error prone or high risk regarding patient safety is measured and analyzed?

b. Do the leaders ensure that when significant variation is identified, appropriate corrective actions are taken to enhance the system(s)?

Score 1   a. and b. Always

Score 2   a. and b.   Usually
Score 3   a. and b.   Sometimes
Score 4   a. and b.   Rarely
Score 5   a. and b.   Never

Standards

LD.4.4   *The leaders allocate adequate resources for measuring, assessing, and improving the hospital's performance and for improving patient safety.*

LD.4.4.1   The leaders assign personnel needed to participate in performance-improvement activities and activities to improve patient safety.

LD.4.4.2   The leaders provide adequate time for personnel to participate in performance-improvement activities and activities to improve patient safety.

LD.4.4.3   The leaders provide information systems and data management processes for ongoing performance improvement and improvement of patient safety.

LD.4.4.4   The leaders provide for staff training in the basic approaches to and methods of performance improvement and improvement of patient safety.

LD.4.4.5   The leaders assess the adequacy of their allocation of human, information, physical, and financial resources in support of their identified performance improvement and safety improvement priorities.

Intent of LD.4.4 Through LD.4.4.5

Hospital leaders provide adequate human resources for these activities and give them sufficient time and support to be effective. Appropriate staff members are assigned in sufficient numbers to ensure progress in the pursuit of improvement priorities and risk-reduction priorities. Leaders allow enough time for performance-improvement activities and activities to improve patient safety and provide needed information and technical assistance. Each department determines what resources are sufficient for its improvement efforts and activities to improve patient safety.

Standard

LD.4.5   The leaders measure and assess the effectiveness of their contributions to improving performance and improving patient safety.

Intent of LD.4.5

The performance-improvement framework in the "Improving Organization Performance" chapter is used to design, measure, assess, and improve the leaders' performance and contribution to performance improvement and improvement in patient safety.

   The leaders
- set measurable objectives for improving hospital performance and improving patient safety;
- gather information to assess their effectiveness in improving hospital performance and in improving patient safety;
- use pre-established, objective process criteria to assess their effectiveness in improving hospital performance and in improving patient safety;
- draw conclusions based on their findings and develop and implement improvement in their activities; and
- evaluate their performance to support sustained improvement.

Scoring for LD.4.4.5

Do the leaders assess the adequacy of their allocation of resources in support of their identified performance improvement and risk reduction priorities?

Score 1   Always
Score 2   Usually
Score 3   Sometimes
Score 4   Rarely
Score 5   Never

1 2 3 4 5 NA

Introduction to Patient Safety and Medical/Health Care Errors Reduction Standards

Standards throughout this manual are designed to improve patient safety and reduce risk to patients. Recognizing that effective medical/health care error reduction requires an integrated and coordinated approach, the following standards relate specifically to leadership's role in an organizationwide safety program that includes all activities within the organization which contribute to the maintenance and improvement of patient safety, such as performance improvement, environmental safety, and risk management. The standards do not require the creation of new structures or "offices" within the organization; rather, the standards emphasize the need to integrate all patient-safety activities, both existing and newly created, with an identified locus of accountability within the organization's leadership.

Although the standards focus on patient safety, it would be difficult to create an organizationwide safety initiative that excludes staff and visitors. Furthermore, many of the activities taken to improve patient safety (e.g., security, equipment safety, infection control) encompass staff and visitors as well as patients.

Effective reduction of medical/health care errors and other factors that contribute to unintended adverse patient outcomes in a health care organization requires an environment in which patients, their families, and organization staff and leaders can identify and manage actual and potential risks to patient safety. This environment encourages recognition and acknowledgment of risks to patient safety and medical/health care errors; the initiation of actions to reduce these risks; the internal reporting of what has been found and the actions taken; a focus on processes and systems; and minimization of individual blame or retribution for involvement in a medical/health care error. It encourages organizational learning about medical/health care errors and supports the sharing of that knowledge to effect behavioral changes in itself and other health care organizations to improve patient safety. The leaders of the organization are responsible for fostering such an environment through their personal example and by establishing mechanisms that support effective responses to actual occurrences; ongoing proactive reduction in medical/health care errors; and integration of patient safety priorities into the new design and redesign of all relevant organization processes, functions, and services.

Standard

LD.5 The leaders ensure implementation of an integrated patient safety program throughout the organization.

Intent of LD.5

The patient safety program includes at least the following:

- Designation of one or more qualified individuals or an interdisciplinary group to manage the organizationwide patient safety program. Typically these individuals may include directors of performance improvement, safety officers, risk managers, and clinical leaders.
- Definition of the scope of the program activities, that is, the types of occurrences to be addressed—typically ranging from "no harm" frequently occurring "slips" to sentinel events with serious adverse outcomes.
- Description of mechanisms to ensure that all components of the health care organization are integrated into and participate in the organizationwide program.
- Procedures for immediate response to medical/health care errors, including care of the affected patient(s), containment of risk to others, and preservation of factual information for subsequent analysis.
- Clear systems for internal and external reporting of information relating to medical/health care errors.
- Defined mechanisms for responding to the various types of occurrences, e.g., root cause analysis in response to a sentinel event, or for conducting proactive risk reduction activities.
- Defined mechanisms for support of staff who have been involved in a sentinel event.
- At least annually, a report to the governing body on the occurrence of medical/health care errors and actions taken to improve patient safety, both in response to actual occurrences and proactively.

Standard

LD.5.1 *Leaders ensure that the processes for identifying and managing sentinel events* are defined and implemented.*

Intent of LD.5.1

When a sentinel event occurs in a health care organization, it is necessary that appropriate individuals within the organization be aware of the event; investigate and understand the causes that underlie the event; and make changes in the organization's systems and processes to reduce the probability of such an event in the future. The leaders are responsible for establishing processes for the identification, reporting, analysis, and prevention of sentinel events and for ensuring the consistent and effective implementation of a mechanism to accomplish these activities including

* sentinel event An unexpected occurrence involving death or serious physical or psychological injury or the risk thereof. Serious injury specifically includes loss of limb or function. The phrase "or risk thereof" includes any process variation for which a recurrence would carry a significant chance of a serious adverse outcome.

- determination of a definition of *sentinel event* and *near misses,* * which are approved by the leaders and communicated throughout the organization; at a minimum, the organization's definition must include those events that are subject to review under the Joint Commission's Sentinel Event Policy;
- creation of a process for reporting of sentinel events through established channels within the organization and, as appropriate, to external agencies in accordance with law and regulation;
- creation of a process for conducting thorough and credible root cause analyses that focus on process and system factors; and
- documentation of a risk-reduction strategy and action plan that includes measurement of the effectiveness of process and system improvements to reduce risk.

Standard

LD.5.2 Leaders ensure that an ongoing, proactive program for identifying risks to patient safety and reducing medical/health care errors is defined and implemented.

Intent of LD.5.2

The organization seeks to reduce the risk of sentinel events and medical/health care system error-related occurrences by conducting its own proactive risk assessment activities and by using available information about sentinel events known to occur in health care organizations that provide similar care and services. This effort is undertaken so that processes, functions, and services can be designed or redesigned to prevent such occurrences in the organization.

Proactive identification and management of potential risks to patient safety have the obvious advantage of *preventing* adverse occurrences, rather than simply *reacting* when they occur. This approach also avoids the barriers to understanding created by hindsight bias and the fear of disclosure, embarrassment, blame, and punishment that can arise in the wake of an actual event.

Leaders provide direction and resources to conduct the following proactive activities to reduce risk to patients:

- At least annually, select at least one high-risk process for proactive risk assessment; such selection is to be based, in part, on information published periodically by the Joint Commission that identifies the most frequently occurring types of sentinel events and patient safety risk factors.
- Assess the intended and actual implementation of the process to identify the steps in the process where there is, or may be, undesirable variation (i.e., what engineers call potential "failure modes").
- For each identified "failure mode" identify the possible effects on patients (what engineers call the "effect"), and how serious the possible effect on the patient could be (what engineers call the "criticality" of the effect).
- For the most critical effects, conduct a root cause analysis to determine why the variation (the failure mode) leading to that effect may occur.
- Redesign the process and/or underlying systems to minimize the risk of that failure mode or to protect patients from the effects of that failure mode.
- Test and implement the redesigned process.
- Identify and implement measures of the effectiveness of the redesigned process.
- Implement a strategy for maintaining the effectiveness of the redesigned process over time.

Standard

LD.5.3 Leaders ensure that patient safety issues are given a high priority and addressed when processes, functions, or services are designed or redesigned.

Intent of LD.5.3

When processes, functions, or services are designed or redesigned, information from within the organization and from other organizations about potential risks to patient safety, including the occurrence of sentinel events, is considered and, where appropriate, used to minimize the risk to patients affected by the new or redesigned process, function, or service.

Scoring for LD.5

1 2 3 4 5 NA

a. Does the patient safety program include designation of one or more qualified individuals or an interdisciplinary group to manage the organizationwide patient safety program?
b. Does the patient safety program include a definition of the scope of the program activities, as described in the intent?
c. Does the patient safety program include a description of mechanisms to ensure that all components of the health care organization are integrated into and participate in the organizationwide program?

* near miss Used to describe any process variation which did not affect the outcome, but for which a recurrence carries a significant chance of a serious adverse outcome. Such a near miss falls within the scope of the definition of a sentinel event, but outside the scope of those sentinel events that are subject to review by the Joint Commission under its Sentinel Event Policy.

d. Does the patient safety program include procedures for immediate response to medical/health care errors, including care of the affected patient(s), containment of risk to others, and preservation of factual information for subsequent analysis?

e. Does the patient safety program include clear systems for internal and external reporting of information relating to medical/health care errors?

f. Does the patient safety program include defined mechanisms for responding to the various types of occurrences, e.g., root cause analysis in response to a sentinel event, or for conducting proactive risk reduction activities?

g. Does the patient safety program include defined mechanisms for support of staff who have been involved in a sentinel event?

h. Is there evidence of a report to the governing body on the occurrence of medical/health care errors and actions taken to improve patient safety, both in response to actual occurrences and proactively at least annually?

Score 1   a. through h. Always

Score 2   a. through h. Usually

Score 3   a. through h. Sometimes

Score 4   a. through h. Rarely

Score 5   a. through h. Never

1 2 3 4 5 NA

Scoring for LD.5.1

a. Have the leaders established processes for identifying and managing sentinel events and near misses as identified in the intent?

b. Have the processes been implemented?

Score 1   a. and b. Yes

Score 3   a. and b. Not consistently

Score 5   a. and b. No

1 2 3 4 5 NA

Scoring for LD.5.2

a. Do the leaders provide direction and resources to prioritize processes that are identified as high risk with respect to patient safety?

b. Do the leaders provide direction and resources to select at least one high-risk process for proactive risk assessment, such selection to be based, in part, on information published periodically by the Joint Commission that identifies the most frequently occurring types of sentinel events and patient safety risk factors, at least annually?

c. Do the leaders provide direction and resources to assess the intended and actual implementation of the process to identify the steps in the process where there is, or may be, undesirable variation?

d. Do the leaders provide direction and resources to identify the possible effects on patients (what engineers call the "effect"), and how serious the possible effect on the patient could be (what engineers call the "criticality" of the effect) for each identified "failure mode"?

e. Do the leaders provide direction and resources to conduct a root cause analysis to determine why the variation (the failure mode) leading to that effect may occur for the most critical effects?

f. Do the leaders provide direction and resources to redesign the process and/or underlying systems to minimize the risk of that failure mode or to protect patients from the effects of that failure mode?

g. Do the leaders provide direction and resources to test and implement the redesigned processes?

h. Do the leaders provide direction and resources to identify and implement measures of the effectiveness of the redesigned process?

i. Do the leaders provide direction and resources to implement a strategy for maintaining the effectiveness of the redesigned process over time?

Score 1   a. through i. Always

Score 2   a. through i. Usually

Score 3   a. through i. Sometimes

Score 4   a. through i Rarely

Score 5   a. through i. Never

Scoring for LD.5.3

This standard is scored at PI.2.

Management of Human Resources (HR)

Standard

HR.4 An orientation process provides initial job training and information and assesses the staff's ability to fulfill specified responsibilities.

Intent of HR.4

The orientation process assesses each staff member's ability to fulfill specific responsibilities. The process familiarizes staff members with their jobs and with the work environment before the staff begins patient care or other activities. In this way, the process promotes safe and effective job performance. The orientation process emphasizes specific job-related aspects of patient safety. When the hospital uses volunteer services, volunteers are oriented to patient care, safety, infection control, and any other activities they are expected to perform competently.

Scoring for HR.4

Have all staff members completed an orientation to promote safe and effective job performance?

1 2 3 4 5 NA

Score 1   90% to 100% compliance

Score 3   80% to 89% compliance

Score 5   Less than 80% compliance

Standard

HR.4.2 Ongoing in-service and other education and training maintain and improve staff competence and support an interdisciplinary approach to patient care.

Intent of HR.4.2

The hospital ensures that each staff member participates in ongoing in-service education and other training to increase his or her knowledge of work-related issues. Ongoing in-service and other education and training programs emphasize specific job-related aspects of patient safety. As appropriate, this training incorporates methods of team training to foster an interdisciplinary, collaborative approach to the delivery of patient care, and reinforces the need and way(s) to report medical/health care errors. The hospital periodically reviews the staff's abilities to carry out job responsibilities, especially when introducing new procedures, techniques, technology, and equipment. Ongoing in-service and other education and training programs are appropriate to patient age groups served by the hospital.

Scoring for HR.4.2

Do staff members participate in an ongoing in-service or other educational program designed to increase their knowledge of work-related issues including patient safety and their ability to carry out job responsibilities, especially when introducing new procedures, techniques, technology, and equipment?

1 2 3 4 5 NA

Score 1   90% to 100% compliance

Score 2   75% to 89% compliance

Score 3   50% to 74% compliance

Score 4   25% to 49% compliance

Score 5   Less than 25% compliance

Management of Information (IM)

Standard

IM.1 The hospital plans and designs information management processes to meet internal and external information needs.

Intent of IM.1

Hospitals vary in size, complexity, governance, structure, decision-making processes, and resources. Information management systems and processes vary accordingly. An information system consists of effective methodologies to maintain and process data. Although computer-based information is often referenced when considering information processing and management, it is understood that data also consist of written, pictorial, graphic, and spoken forms, for which information management systems are used to manage and continuously improve care and organizational processes.

The hospital bases its information management processes on a thorough analysis of internal and external information needs. The analysis ascertains the flow of information in a hospital, including information storage and feedback mechanisms. The analysis considers what data and information are needed within and among departments, services, or programs, the clinical staff, the administration, and governance structure, as well as information needed to support relationships with outside services, contractors, companies, and agencies. The hospital bases management, staffing, and material resource allocations for information management on the scope and complexity of services provided. Leaders seek input from staff in information needs, selecting appropriate information technology, and integrating and using information systems to manage clinical and organizational information. Appropriate staff and leaders ensure that required data and information are provided efficiently for individual care, research, education, and management at every level.

The hospital assesses its information management needs based on its

- mission;
- goals;
- services;
- personnel;
- mode(s) of service delivery;
- resources;
- access to affordable technology; and
- identification of barriers to effective communication among caregivers.

The hospital also considers its information needs for

- licensing, accrediting, and regulatory bodies;
- purchasers, payers, and employers; and
- participation in national research and care databases.

This analysis guides development of processes for managing information used internally and externally.

When the hospital assesses its overall information needs, it also looks at the need for knowledge-based information. The hospital's services, resources, and systems for knowledge-based information are based on a thorough needs assessment, which addresses

- the needs of those who will use the information;
- accessibility and timeliness;
- links with the hospital's internal information systems; and
- links with external databases and information networks.

1 2 3 4 5 NA

Scoring for IM.1

a. Is the design of information management processes based on a comprehensive assessment of needs that considers the elements listed in the intent?

b. Are internal and external information management processes appropriate for the hospital's size and complexity?

c. Does the hospital base management, staffing, and material resource allocations for information management on the scope and complexity of services provided?

d. Do appropriate staff members participate in assessing, selecting, integrating, and using information management systems for clinical and organizational information?

Score 1   a. through d. Always

Score 2   a. through d. Usually

Score 3   a. through d. Sometimes

Score 4   a. through d. Rarely

Score 5   a. through d. Never

Standard

IM.5 Transmission of data and information is timely and accurate.

Intent of IM.5

Internally and externally generated data and information are accurately transmitted to users. The integrity of data and information is maintained, and adequate communication exists between data users and suppliers. Specific attention is directed to the processes for ensuring accurate, timely, and complete verbal and written communication among care givers and all others involved in the utilization of data. The timing of transmission is appropriate to the data's intended use.

Scoring for IM.5

Is the transmission of data and information timely and accurate, as appropriate for its intended use and as defined by user needs?

Score 1   Always

Score 2   Usually

Score 3   Sometimes

Score 4   Rarely

Score 5   Never

1 2 3 4 5 NA

Standards

IM.7 *The hospital defines, captures, analyzes, transforms, transmits, and reports patient-specific data and information related to care processes and outcomes.*

IM.7.1 The hospital initiates and maintains a medical record for every individual assessed or treated.

IM.7.1.1 Only authorized individuals make entries in medical records.

IM.7.1.2 The hospital determines how long medical record information is retained, based on law and regulation and the information use for patient care, legal, research, and educational purposes.

IM.7.2 The medical record contains sufficient information to identify the patient, support the diagnosis, justify the treatment, document the course and results, and promote continuity of care among health care providers.

Intent of IM.7 Through IM.7.2

Information management processes provide for the use of patient-specific data and information to

- facilitate patient care;
- serve as a financial and legal record;
- aid in clinical research;
- support decision analysis; and
- guide professional and organizational performance improvement.

To facilitate consistency and continuity in patient care, specific data and information are required. Administrative and direct patient care providers produce and use this information for professional and organization improvement. Medical records contain sufficient information to

- identify the patient;
- support the diagnosis;
- justify the treatment;
- document the course and results; and
- facilitate continuity of care.

The environment in which patient-specific information is provided supports timely, accurate, secure, and confidential recording and use of patient-specific information. The system recalls historical patient data and is able to furnish data about current encounters. To facilitate consistency and continuity in patient care, the medical record contains very specific data and information, including

a.   the patient's name, address, date of birth, and the name of any legally authorized representative;

b.   the legal status of patients receiving mental health services;

c.   emergency care provided to the patient prior to arrival, if any;

d.   the record and findings of the patient's assessment;

e.   conclusions or impressions drawn from the medical history and physical examination;

f.   the diagnosis or diagnostic impression;

g.   the reasons for admission or treatment;

h.   the goals of treatment and the treatment plan;

i.   evidence of known advance directives;

j.   evidence of informed consent, when required by hospital policy;

k.   diagnostic and therapeutic orders, if any;

l.   all diagnostic and therapeutic procedures and test results;

m.   test results relevant to the management of the patient's condition;

n. all operative and other invasive procedures performed, using acceptable disease and operative terminology that includes etiology, as appropriate;

o. progress notes made by the medical staff and other authorized individuals;

p. all reassessments and any revisions of the treatment plan;

q. clinical observations;

r. the patient's response to care;

s. consultation reports;

t. every medication ordered or prescribed for an inpatient;

u. every medication dispensed to an ambulatory patient or an inpatient on discharge;

v. every dose of medication administered and any adverse drug reaction;

w. all relevant diagnoses established during the course of care;

x. any referrals and communications made to external or internal care providers and to community agencies;

y. conclusions at termination of hospitalization;

z. discharge instructions to the patient and family; and

aa. clinical résumés and discharge summaries, or a final progress note or transfer summary.

A concise clinical résumé included in the medical record at discharge provides important information to other caregivers and facilitates continuity of care. For patients discharged to ambulatory (outpatient) care, the clinical résumé summarizes previous levels of care. The discharge summary contains the following information:

- The reason for hospitalization;
- Significant findings;
- Procedures performed and treatment rendered;
- The patient's condition at discharge; and
- Instructions to the patient and family, if any.

For newborns with uncomplicated deliveries, or for patients hospitalized for less than 48 hours with only minor problems, a progress note may substituted for the clinical résumé. The medical staff defines what problems and interventions may be considered minor. The progress note, which may be handwritten, documents the patient's condition at discharge, discharge instructions, and required follow-up care.

When a patient is transferred within the same organization from one level of care to another (for example, from the hospital to residential care), and the caregivers change, a transfer summary may be substituted for the clinical résumé. A transfer summary briefly describes the patient's condition at time of transfer, and the reason for the transfer. When the caregivers remain the same, a progress note may suffice.

1 2 3 4 5 NA

Scoring for IM.7.1

Does the hospital initiate and maintain, for all patients it treats in any setting, medical records containing all items listed in the intent?

Score 1 Yes

Score 5 No

1 2 3 4 5 NA

Scoring for IM.7.1.1

Are policies followed regarding authorization to make entries in the medical record?

Score 1 Always

Score 2 Usually

Score 3 Sometimes

Score 4 Rarely

Score 5 Never

OR

No such policies exist.

1 2 3 4 5 NA

Scoring for IM.7.1.2

a. Does the hospital have a policy on keeping medical records information, as described in the standard?

b. Is the policy followed?

Score 1 a. Yes

b. Always

Score 2 b. Usually

Score 3 b. Sometimes

Score 4   b.   Rarely

Score 5   a.   No

b.   Never

Scoring for IM.7.2

1 2 3 4 5 NA

What percentage of medical records contains sufficient information to

- identify the patient;
- support the diagnosis;
- justify the treatment;
- document the course and results; and
- facilitate continuity of care?

Score 1   90% to 100% of those reviewed

Score 2   75% to 89% of those reviewed

Score 3   50% to 74% of those reviewed

Score 4   25% to 49% of those reviewed

Score 5   Less than 25% of those reviewed

Standard

IM.8 The hospital collects and aggregates data and information to support care and service delivery and operations.

Intent of IM.8

Certain types of data and information need to be accumulated over time to support the hospital's clinical and management functions. The hospital assesses its need for aggregated data and information and defines the types of required data and information. The information management function has the ability to collect and aggregate clinical and administrative data to support

- individual care and care delivery;
- decision making;
- management and operations;
- analysis of trends over time;
- performance comparisons over time within the hospital and with other hospitals;
- performance improvement; and
- reduction in risks to patients.

The hospital is able to aggregate the data and information requirements specified in this manual, as well as identified indicator data for performance measurement.

Scoring for IM.8

1 2 3 4 5 NA

Does the hospital collect and aggregate data to support the functions in this manual and the hospital's assessed needs?

Score 1   Always

Score 2   Usually

Score 3   Sometimes

Score 4   Rarely

Score 5   Never

Standard

IM.9 Knowledge-based information systems, resources, and services meet the hospital's needs.

Intent of IM.9

Appropriate knowledge-based information is acquired, assembled, and transmitted to users. Knowledge-based information management consists of systems, resources, and services to

- help health professionals acquire and maintain the knowledge and skills they need to maintain and improve competence;
- support clinical and management decision making;

- support performance improvement and activities to reduce risk to patients;
- provide needed information and education to individuals and families; and
- satisfy research-related needs.
    Knowledge-based information refers to current authoritative print and nonprint information resources, including
- current periodicals, indexes, and abstracts in print or electronic format;
- other clinical and managerial literature;
- successful practices;
- practice guidelines;
- research data;
- recent editions of texts and other resources;
- satellite television services; and
- on-line computer-linked information services via the Internet.

1 2 3 4 5 NA

Scoring for IM.9

a. Does the hospital have a plan that identifies the need for clinical and managerial literature, successful practices, reference information, and research data and information?

b. Does the hospital provide clinical and managerial literature, successful practices, reference information, and research data to meet its identified needs as outlined in its plan?

Score 1   a. Yes
           b. Always

Score 2   b. Usually

Score 3   a. No
           b. Sometimes

Score 4   b. Rarely

Score 5   b. Never

Index

How Well Does *Front Line of Defense: The Role of Nurses in Preventing Sentinel Events* Meet Your Needs?

We would like to know your opinion of *Front Line of Defense: The Role of Nurses in Preventing Sentinel Events*. Your comments are important; they help us evaluate and improve our publications to better meet your needs. Please take a few minutes to complete and mail this postage-paid card.

Please indicate whether you agree or disagree with the following statements:	Strongly Agree	Agree	Somewhat Agree	Somewhat Disagree	Strongly Disagree
■ *Front Line of Defense: The Role of Nurses in Preventing Sentinel Events* provides useful and timely information.	❏	❏	❏	❏	❏
■ *Front Line of Defense: The Role of Nurses in Preventing Sentinel Events* presents new concepts/ practical strategies for prevention of sentinel events and near misses.	❏	❏	❏	❏	❏
■ *Front Line of Defense: The Role of Nurses in Preventing Sentinel Events* is a value for its price.	❏	❏	❏	❏	❏
■ I would recommend *Front Line of Defense: The Role of Nurses in Preventing Sentinel Events* to a colleague.	❏	❏	❏	❏	❏

Please rate the value of the following elements:	Extremely Valuable	Very Valuable	Somewhat Valuable	Not Very Valuable	Not at all Valuable
■ Overall Design	❏	❏	❏	❏	❏
■ Introduction	❏	❏	❏	❏	❏
■ Chapter 1: Preventing Operative and Preoperative Errors and Complications	❏	❏	❏	❏	❏
■ Chapter 2: Preventing Medication Errors	❏	❏	❏	❏	❏
■ Chapter 3: Preventing Transfusion Errors	❏	❏	❏	❏	❏
■ Chapter 4: Preventing Falls	❏	❏	❏	❏	❏
■ Chapter 5: Preventing Infant Abductions and Release to Wrong Families	❏	❏	❏	❏	❏
■ Chapter 6: Preventing Serious Injury or Death in Physical Restraints	❏	❏	❏	❏	❏
■ Chapter 7: Preventing Serious Injury or Death Following Elopement	❏	❏	❏	❏	❏
■ Chapter 8: Preventing Suicide	❏	❏	❏	❏	❏
■ Chapter 9: Preventing Treatment Delays	❏	❏	❏	❏	❏
■ Chapter 10: Concluding Comments	❏	❏	❏	❏	❏
■ Selected Resources	❏	❏	❏	❏	❏
■ Appendix: Safety and Health Care Error Reduction Standards	❏	❏	❏	❏	❏
■ Other (please be specific) _____	❏	❏	❏	❏	❏

I will use *Front Line of Defense: The Role of Nurses in Preventing Sentinel Events* to (please check all that apply):

❏ Identify how I can improve my own personal performance within the health care system.
❏ Help facilitate organizationwide ongoing error prevention and performance improvement.
❏ Educate staff on prevention techniques.
❏ Other (please be specific)_____ .

Please make additional comments about *Front Line of Defense: The Role of Nurses in Preventing Sentinel Events*:

_____
_____

Characteristics of my organization:
My job title is: _____
■ Type of organization:_____
■ Size: ❏ Small ❏ Medium ❏ Large
■ State(s) in which your organization operates: _____
■ Other health care entities affiliated with your organization (such as long term care, home care, etc):
_____

If we may contact you for additional feedback about this or any other Joint Commission Resources publication or for suggestions for future publications, please provide the following information:
Name: _____
Organization: _____
Address:_____
Telephone number: (____)_____
E-mail: _____

If you would like more information about Joint Commission Resources publications, please call our Customer Service Center at 630/792-5800. Our Customer Service Center is open from 8:00 AM to 5:00 PM central standard time, Monday through Friday.
Thank you!

BUSINESS REPLY MAIL

FIRST CLASS MAIL   PERMIT NO 632   VILLA PARK IL

POSTAGE WILL BE PAID BY ADDRESSEE

Attn: Kim Andersen
Joint Commission Resources
One Renaissance Boulevard
Oakbrook Terrace IL 60181-9887